BRAIN METASTASES

Cancer Treatment and Research
Steven T. Rosen, M.D., *Series Editor*

Pienta, K.J. (ed.): *Diagnosis and Treatment of Genitourinary Malignancies.* 1996. ISBN 0-7923-4164-3.
Arnold, A.J. (ed.): *Endocrine Neoplasms.* 1997. ISBN 0-7923-4354-9.
Pollock, R.E. (ed.): *Surgical Oncology.* 1997. ISBN 0-7923-9900-5.
Verweij, J., Pinedo, H.M., Suit, H.D. (eds): *Soft Tissue Sarcomas: Present Achievements and Future Prospects.* 1997. ISBN 0-7923-9913-7.
Walterhouse, D.O., Cohn, S. L. (eds): *Diagnostic and Therapeutic Advances in Pediatric Oncology.* 1997. ISBN 0-7923-9978-1.
Mittal, B.B., Purdy, J.A., Ang, K.K. (eds): *Radiation Therapy.* 1998. ISBN 0-7923-9981-1.
Foon, K.A., Muss, H.B. (eds): *Biological and Hormonal Therapies of Cancer.* 1998. ISBN 0-7923-9997-8.
Ozols, R.F. (ed.): *Gynecologic Oncology.* 1998. ISBN 0-7923-8070-3.
Noskin, G. A. (ed.): *Management of Infectious Complications in Cancer Patients.* 1998. ISBN 0-7923-8150-5.
Bennett, C. L. (ed.): *Cancer Policy.* 1998. ISBN 0-7923-8203-X.
Benson, A. B. (ed.): *Gastrointestinal Oncology.* 1998. ISBN 0-7923-8205-6.
Tallman, M.S., Gordon, L.I. (eds): *Diagnostic and Therapeutic Advances in Hematologic Malignancies.* 1998. ISBN 0-7923-8206-4.
von Gunten, C.F. (ed.): *Palliative Care and Rehabilitation of Cancer Patients.* 1999. ISBN 0-7923-8525-X.
Burt, R.K., Brush, M.M. (eds): *Advances in Allogeneic Hematopoietic Stem Cell Transplantation.* 1999. ISBN 0-7923-7714-1.
Angelos, P. (ed.): *Ethical Issues in Cancer Patient Care* 2000. ISBN 0-7923-7726-5.
Gradishar, W.J., Wood, W.C. (eds): *Advances in Breast Cancer Management.* 2000. ISBN 0-7923-7890-3.
Sparano, J. A. (ed.): *HIV & HTLV-I Associated Malignancies.* 2001. ISBN 0-7923-7220-4.
Ettinger, D. S. (ed.): *Thoracic Oncology.* 2001. ISBN 0-7923-7248-4.
Bergan, R. C. (ed.): *Cancer Chemoprevention.* 2001. ISBN 0-7923-7259-X.
Raza, A., Mundle, S.D. (eds): *Myelodysplastic Syndromes & Secondary Acute Myelogenous Leukemia* 2001. ISBN 0-7923-7396.
Talamonti, M. S. (ed.): *Liver Directed Therapy for Primary and Metastatic Liver Tumors.* 2001. ISBN 0-7923-7523-8.
Stack, M.S., Fishman, D.A. (eds). *Ovarian Cancer.* 2001. ISBN 0-7923-7530-0
Bashey, A., Ball, E.D. (eds): *Non-Myeloablative Allogeneic Transplantation.* 2002. ISBN 0-7923-7646-3.
Leong, S. P.L. (ed.): *Atlas of Selective Sentinel Lymphadenectomy for Melanoma, Breast Cancer and Colon Cancer.* 2002. ISBN 1-4020-7013-6.
Andersson , B., Murray D. (eds): *Clinically Relevant Resistance in Cancer Chemotherapy.* 2002. ISBN 1-4020-7200-7.
Beam, C. (ed.): *Biostatistical Applications in Cancer Research.* 2002. ISBN 1-4020-7226-0.
Brockstein, B., Masters, G. (eds): *Head and Neck Cancer.* 2003. ISBN 1-4020-7336-4.
Frank, D.A. (ed.): *Signal Transduction in Cancer.* 2003. ISBN 1-4020-7340-2.
Figlin, R. A. (ed.): *Kidney Cancer.* 2003. ISBN 1-4020-7457-3.
Kirsch, M.; Black, P. McL. (ed.): *Angiogenesis in Brain Tumors.* 2003. ISBN 1-4020-7704-1.
Keller, E.T., Chung, L.W.K. (eds): *The Biology of Skeletal Metastases.* 2004. ISBN 1-4020-7749-1.
Kumar, R. (ed.): *Molecular Targeting and Signal Transduction.* 2004. ISBN 1-4020-7822-6.
Verweij, J., Pinedo, H.M. (eds): *Targeting Treatment of Soft Tissue Sarcomas.* 2004. ISBN 1-4020-7808-0.
Finn, W.G., Peterson, L.C. (eds.): *Hematopathology in Oncology.* 2004. ISBN 1-4020-7919-2.
Farid, N. (ed.): *Molecular Basis of Thyroid Cancer.* 2004. ISBN 1-4020-8106-5.
Khleif, S. (ed.): *Tumor Immunology and Cancer* Vaccines. 2004. ISBN 1-4020-8119-7.
Balducci, L., Extermann, M. (eds): *Biological Basis of Geriatric Oncology.* 2004. ISBN
Abrey, L.E., Chamberlain, M.C., Engelhard, H.H. (eds): *Leptomeningeal Metastases.* 2005. ISBN 0-387-24198-1
Platanias, L.C. (ed.): *Cytokines and Cancer.* 2005. ISBN 0-387-24360-7.
Leong, S.P.L., Kitagawa, Y., Kitajima, M. (eds): *Selective Sentinel Lymphadenectomy for Human Solid Cancer.* 2005. ISBN 0-387-23603-1.
Small, Jr. W., Woloschak, G. (eds): *Radiation Toxicity: A Practical Guide.* 2005. ISBN 1-4020-8053-0.
Haefner, B., Dalgleish, A. (eds): *The Link Between Inflammation and Cancer.* 2006. ISBN 0-387-26282-2.
Leonard, J.P., Coleman, M. (eds): *Hodgkin's and Non-Hodgkin's Lymphoma.* 2006. ISBN 0-387-29345.
Leong, S.P.L. (ed): *Cancer Clinical Trials: Proactive Strategies.* 2006. ISBN 0-387-33224-3.
Meyers, C. (ed): *Aids-Associated Viral Oncogenesis.* 2007. ISBN 978-0-387-46804-4.
Ceelen, W.P. (ed): *Peritoneal Carcinomatosis: A Multidisciplinary Approach.* 2007. ISBN 978-0-387-48991-9.
Leong, S.P.L. (ed): *Cancer Metastasis and the Lymphovascular System: Basis for rational therapy.* 2007. ISBN 978-0-387-69218-0.
Raizer, J., Abrey, L.E. (eds): *Brain Metastases.* 2007. ISBN 978-0-387-69221-0.

BRAIN METASTASES

edited by

Jeffrey J. Raizer, MD
Director, Medical Neuro-Oncology.
Department of Neurology
Robert H. Lurie Comprehensive Cancer Center
Northwestern University, Feinberg School of Medicine
Chicago, Illinois, USA

Lauren E. Abrey, MD
Director of Clinical Research
Department of Neurology
Memorial Sloan-Kettering Cancer Center
New York, New York, USA

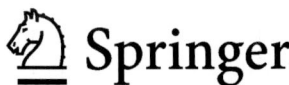 Springer

Jeffrey J. Raizer, MD
Northwestern University, Feinberg School of Medicine
Robert H. Lurie Comprehensive Cancer Center
Department of Neurology
Chicago, IL 60611

Lauren E. Abrey, MD
Memorial Sloan-Kettering Cancer Center
Department of Neurology
1275 York Avenue
New York, NY 10021

Series Editor:
Steven T. Rosen
Robert H. Lurie Comprehensive Cancer Center
Northwestern University
Chicago, IL
USA

Brain Metastases

Library of Congress Control Number: 2006939125

ISBN 978-0-387-69221-0   e-ISBN 978-0-387-69222-7

Printed on acid-free paper.

Contents

Contributors... vii

Introduction.. xi

Acknowledgments... xiii

1. Brain Metastases: Epidemiology and Pathophysiology............... 1
   Joohee Sul and Jerome B. Posner

2. The Economics of Brain Metastases 23
   Charles L. Bennett MD PhD MPP, Cara C. Tigue BA,
   and Karen A. Fitzner PhD

3. Neuroimaging of Parenchymal Brain Metastases.................... 31
   Matthew T. Walker, MD and Vipul Kapoor, MD

4. Symptom Management and Supportive Care
   of the Patient with Brain Metastases 53
   Herbert B. Newton, M.D., FAAN

5. Surgery for Brain Metastases 75
   Sunit Das M.D., Ph.D, Kenji Muro M.D. and Jeffrey J. Raizer M.D.

6. Radiation for Brain Metastases.................................... 91
   Malika L. Siker, M.D. and Minesh P. Mehta, M.D.

7. Dural and Skull Base Metastases 117
   Arnaldo Neves Da Silva, M.D. and David Schiff, M.D.

8. Pediatric Brain Metastasis from Extraneural
   Malignancies: A Review... 143
   Stewart Goldman, MD, María E. Echevarría,
   MD, Jason Fangusaro, MD

9. Brain Metastases in Hematologic Malignancies 169
   Nancy D. Doolittle, Ph.D.

10. Chemotherapy for Brain Metastases: Breast, Gynecologic
    and Non-Melanoma Skin Malignancies 185
    Gaurav D. Shah, MD and Lauren E. Abrey, MD

**11. Chemotherapy for Brain Metastases
    due to Lung Cancer and Melanoma** **199**
    Marc C Chamberlain, M.D.

12. Palliative Care for Patients With Brain Metastases **215**
    Keren Barfi, M.D., Herbert Newton M.D.,
    FAAN, Jamie Von Roenn, M.D.

    Subject Index **235**

Contributors

Lauren E. Abrey, MD
Memorial Sloan-Kettering Cancer Center
Department of Neurology
New York, NY 10021

Keren Barfi, MD
Northwestern University
Department of Hematology/Oncology
Chicago, IL 60611

Charles L. Bennett, MD PhD MPP
Division of Hematology/Oncology
Feinberg School of Medicine
The Robert H. Lurie Comprehensive Cancer Center
Northwestern University
Chicago, IL 60611

Marc C. Chamberlain, M.D.
Department of Neurology
University of Washington
Fred Hutchinson Cancer Research Center
Seattle Cancer Care Alliance
825 Eastlake Ave E
Seattle, WA 98109-1023

Arnaldo Neves Da Silva, MD
University of Virginia
Neurology Department, Division of Neuro-Oncology
Charlottesville, VA 22908-0432

Sunit Das, MD, PhD
Department of Neurological Surgery
Northwestern University
Feinberg School of Medicine
Chicago, IL 60611

Nancy D. Doolittle, PhD
Department of Neurology
Oregon Health & Science University
Portland, OR 97239-3098

María E. Echevarría, MD
Children's Memorial Hospital
Division of Hematology/Oncology and Stem Cell Transplantation
Chicago, IL 60611

Jason Fangusaro, MD
Children's Memorial Hospital
Division of Hematology/Oncology and Stem Cell Transplantation
Chicago, IL 60611

Karen A. Fitzner PhD
Division of Hematology/Oncology
Feinberg School of Medicine
The Robert H. Lurie Comprehensive Cancer Center
Northwestern University
Chicago, IL 60611

Stewart Goldman, MD
Children's Memorial Hospital
Division of Hematology/Oncology and Stem Cell Transplantation
Chicago, IL 60611

Vipul Kapoor, MD
Department of Radiology
Feinberg School of Medicine
Chicago, IL 60611

Minesh P. Mehta, MD
University of Wisconsin School of Medicine and Public Health
Department of Human Oncology
Madison, WI 53792

Kenji Muro, MD
Department of Neurological Surgery
Northwestern University
Feinberg School of Medicine
Chicago, IL 60611

Herbert B. Newton, MD, FAAN
Dardinger Neuro-Oncology Center
Department of Neurology
The Ohio State University Hospitals
Columbus, OH 43210

Jerome Posner, MD
Department of Neurology
Memorial Sloan-Kettering Cancer Center
New York, NY 10021

Jeffrey J. Raizer, MD
Department of Neurology
Northwestern University
Feinberg School of Medicine
Chicago, Illinois 60611

David Schiff, MD
University of Virginia
Neurology Department, Division of Neuro-Oncology
Charlottesville, VA 22908-0432

Gaurav D. Shah, MD
Memorial Sloan-Kettering Cancer Center
Department of Neurology
New York, NY 10021

Malika L. Siker, MD
University of Wisconsin School of Medicine and Public Health
Department of Human Oncology
Madison, WI 53792

Joohee Sul
Department of Neurology
Memorial Sloan-Kettering Cancer Center
New York, NY 10021

Cara C. Tigue, BA
Division of Hematology/Oncology
Feinberg School of Medicine
The Robert H. Lurie Comprehensive Cancer Center
Northwestern University
Chicago, IL 60611

Jamie Von Roenn, MD
Northwestern University
Department of Hematology/Oncology
Chicago, IL 60611

Matthew T. Walker, MD
Section Chief of Neuroradiology
Feinberg School of Medicine
Chicago, IL 60611

Introduction

Brain metastases are among the most feared and debilitating complication of systemic cancer. They impact approximately 170 000 patients a year in the United States, a number ten-fold greater than malignant gliomas. Historically, brain metastases were diagnosed in patients with widespread systemic malignancy. Recent improvements in systemic therapies are changing the incidence of brain metastases. More patients are being diagnosed with brain metastases in the setting of controlled systemic tumor.

In this book we provide succinct and up-to-date information to help manage cancer patients who have the misfortune to develop brain metastases. A multidisciplinary assessment involving neurosurgery, radiation oncology, neuro-oncology and medical oncology is critical to optimize patient management and outcome. While average survival remains poor, recent advances in surgery, radiation and chemotherapy may improve disease control and quality of life for many patients.

We hope this book will not only serve as a reference for practitioners in oncology but also stimulate ideas for future research.

Acknowledgments

I want to thank my wife Kelly, my daughter Jordan and my son Adam for their love and support. I want to thank the authors for their efforts in contributing to this book, especially Dr. Jerome Posner for his indispensable contributions to neuro-oncology and for his teachings over the years and to my co-editor Dr. Lauren Abrey for working on this book with me.

   This book is dedicated to them and to all patients who are diagnosed with cancer.

Jeffrey J. Raizer, MD

1. Brain Metastases: Epidemiology and Pathophysiology

Joohee Sul and Jerome B. Posner

Brain metastases are a devastating complication of systemic cancer. Although they typically occur late in the course of the disease, their symptoms of seizures, paralysis and cognitive failure have a major negative impact on quality of life and, once detected, they portend a poor prognosis. Most patients die within months, either from the brain metastasis itself, or if that can be controlled, from widespread systemic disease. Recent data suggest a rise in the incidence of brain metastases [1], so that clinicians face mounting challenges in caring for these patients. New and more effective strategies for the diagnosis and treatment of brain metastases are needed. Development of such strategies will probably require greater knowledge both of the epidemiology and pathophysiology of brain metastases, the topics covered in this chapter.

Epidemiology

Incidence

Brain metastases are almost certainly the most common intracerebral tumor although their exact incidence is not known. [2][3] Primary brain tumors are usually recorded in cancer databases such as Surveillance Epidemiology and End Results (SEER), but there are no national cancer databases that specifically document brain metastases. Epidemiological studies, most of which are outdated, underestimate the incidence of brain metastases. In 1970, Guomundsson published data from Iceland that revealed an annual incidence of 2.8 brain metastases per 100,000 persons. The annual incidence of primary brain tumors during this interval was 7.8 per 100,000 [4]. In a review of records from Olmstead County, Minnesota (Mayo Clinic) over a 33 year period, Percy et al found the incidence of brain metastases to be 11.1 per 100,000, comparable to the rate of primary brain tumors which was 12.5/100,000 [5]. Another retrospective Finnish study, conducted from 1975 to 1985, found the incidence of brain metastases and primary brain tumors to be 3.4/100,000 and 12.3/100,000, respectively [6]. All three authors acknowledged that metastatic brain disease is inadequately captured and the incidence rates are likely higher. There are several reasons for this. Some lesions may have been asymptomatic and consequently escaped clinical detection. In others, particularly those with widespread disease, development of neurologic symptomatology may not have been recognized or may have been ignored, especially in the years before non-invasive brain imaging studies were available. In addition, in patients with multiple metastatic problems, brain metastases may not have been documented in admission and discharge notes.

In 1975, The National Institute of Neurological and Communicative Disorders and Stroke (NINCDS) launched a survey to determine the incidence, prevalence and economic burden of brain tumors in the United States. They identified patients who had been admitted to hospital with a diagnosis of intracranial tumors from 1973–1974. They identified 34,410 patients; 17,030 with primary and 17,380 with metastatic tumors [7]. Of the metastatic tumors, only 3,410 (20%) were histologically verified, compared with 12,610 (74%) of primary tumors. In addition, the discharge diagnoses of "rule out brain tumor", "suspect brain tumor", and "possible brain tumor" were excluded from the analysis, thereby influencing ascertainment.

Although admission and discharge diagnoses and surgical pathologic data reliably identify the incidence of *primary* brain tumors, autopsy studies are better in determining the true prevalence of secondary brain tumors. The prevalence of brain metastases discovered post-mortem is far higher than the prevalence reported in ante-mortem studies. In 1978, Posner and Chernik [8] found intracranial metastases at autopsy in 24% of 2,375 patients who died of cancer; 15% were in the brain parenchyma, 8% in the leptomeninges, and 20% in the dura. They estimated that approximately two-thirds of these lesions had been symptomatic in life [9]. Using these data, Posner estimated that in 1994, 80,000 patients may have had significant neurologic symptomatology due to intracranial metastases during their lifetime [2]. Even if that figure was overestimated by 100%, 40,000 patients with metastatic brain tumors is still more than double the number of primary brain tumors.

In 1983, Pickren et al. reviewed 10,916 autopsy cases and reported 954 (8.7%) instances of intraparenchymal brain metastases [10]. Leptomeningeal and dural metastases were not counted, although many of these are symptomatic. Unfortunately, comprehensive autopsy studies such as this are unlikely to be repeated, because the autopsy rate has dropped precipitously despite the fact that significant errors in clinical diagnosis are still detected. [11]

Many observers believe that the incidence of brain metastases has increased in the United States over the last several decades [12]; however, hard evidence is lacking. An apparent increase in the frequency of brain metastases could result from better ascertainment by more sensitive and less invasive imaging techniques. Such better ascertainment was the primary reason for an apparent increased incidence in primary brain tumors in the 1980s. If the incidence of brain metastases is indeed increasing, it may be due in part to the fact that survival times are longer in most cancers, thereby allowing brain metastases the opportunity to develop [13][14]. According to the American Cancer Society (ACS), the 5-year survival rate for all cancers diagnosed between 1995 and 2001 is 65%, compared with 50% in 1974 to 1976. Surveillance imaging of patients without neurological symptoms is not customarily performed. One exception is in patients with lung cancer. Both non-small cell and small cell histologies have a known propensity to spread to the CNS. Routine brain imaging in these patients has at times led to the detection of asymptomatic lesions [15][16]. As newer techniques such as positron emission tomography (PET) scans become available, it raises the question of whether or not surveillance imaging done with these technologies may reveal an even higher incidence of occult brain metastases. One study from the United Kingdom found that PET scanning detected intracranial disease in 4/273 (1.5%) patients with various malignancies. Of these, two were unsuspected prior to this imaging [17]. Although detection of these lesions may improve our epidemiological data, the clinical significance of these quiescent lesions is often unclear. Conversely, evaluating for systemic disease in a patient with a brain lesion may prove helpful; in roughly 10% of patients, the presence of a brain metastasis leads to the diagnosis of a primary tumor elsewhere [18].

More recently, new indications for surveillance imaging have emerged. Many clinical trials using experimental agents prohibit enrollment of subjects with CNS disease. This has led to an increase in the number of screening MRIs and subsequent detection of occult brain metastases. Since most protocol patients are required to have good functional status, they represent a different population than typical patients who are diagnosed at late stages of disease. As data from these studies are collected, they will be useful in determining the timing and incidence of asymptomatic brain metastases.

Incidence of Brain Metastases from Specific Cancers

Specific types of cancer have a proclivity to spread to the CNS more frequently than others. The most common source of brain metastases is lung cancer [3]. In Posner and Chernik's autopsy review, lung cancer was established as the source of brain metastases in 18-24% of cases [8]. Other tumors that frequently metastasize to the brain include breast, melanoma, colorectal and renal cell cancer. Hematologic malignancies accounted for 10% of metastases, primarily to the leptomeninges [8].

Two recent studies have attempted to identify the incidence of brain metastases clinically or radiologically diagnosed in large cohorts of the patient's cancer (Table 1). In 2004, Barnholtz-Sloan and colleagues [19] analyzed a cohort of 16,210 individuals in the metropolitan Detroit, Michigan vicinity who developed brain metastases from lung, breast, melanoma, renal or colorectal cancer between 1973 to 2001. In this study, the overall frequency of brain metastases from primary tumors was 9.6%. The most common source was lung cancer (19.9%), melanoma (6.9%), renal (6.5%) and breast cancer (5.1%). Only 1.8% of colorectal cancers metastasized to the brain.

Table 1. Incidence of Brain Metastases

Primary Tumor	# (%) of Metastases [19]	#(%) Metastases [21]
Lung	11,763/59,038 (19.9%)	156/938 (16.3%)
Breast	2,635/51,898 (5.1%)	42/802 (5.0%)
Renal	467/7205 (6.5%)	12/114 (9.8%)
Melanoma	566/8229 (6.9%)	12/150 (7.4%)
Colorectal	779/42,817 (1.8%)	10/720 (1.2%)

Another study identified patients [20] diagnosed between 1986 and 1995 with breast cancer, colorectal cancer, lung cancer and renal cancer in a single University Hospital [21]. Patients were followed for up to five years. Brain metastases developed in 16.3% of patients with lung cancer, 9.8% with renal cancer, 7.4% with melanoma, 5% with breast cancer and 1.2% with colorectal cancer.

Although lung cancer constitutes the largest proportion of brain metastases, melanoma, which represents approximately 1% of all cancers, has the greatest propensity to disseminate to the brain. At autopsy, as many as 90% of patients with melanoma exhibit brain metastases [22]. In roughly 80% of patients, the diagnosis of brain metastases is made in patients already known to have cancer (metachronous presentation). Less common is the scenario where the primary and brain metastases are diagnosed simultaneously (synchronous presentation), or the brain disease is discovered first (precocious presentation) [23]. In as many as 15% of patients with precocious brain metastases, the origin of the primary tumor may not be determined [24][25]. If biopsied, the histology is usually adenocarcinoma or poorly differentiated carcinoma of indeterminate origin [26]. If the primary is finally discovered, it is usually from the lung.

Brain metastases occur with equal frequency in men and women. However, when comparing related organs, there are disparities. Both testicular and penile cancers are more likely to metastasize to the brain than are ovarian or vulvar cancer [10]. The age of diagnosis is usually in the 5th to 7th decades of life [14]. This is in accordance with statistics from the American Cancer Society which show that the probability of developing invasive cancer is highest in those ages 60 to 79.

Even within a given primary cancer, some subtypes have a greater propensity to cause brain metastases than others. For example, small-cell lung cancer is more likely to cause brain metastases than non-small cell lung cancer. Younger patients with hormone receptor negative breast cancers suffer more brain metastases [12]. Breast cancers over expressing human epidermal growth factor receptor 2 (HER-2) are more likely to metastasize to brain than are those who are HER-2 negative [27]. Head and neck melanomas are more likely to metastasize to the brain than are melanomas elsewhere [28].

Brain metastases can occur as single or multiple lesions. When a lone brain lesion exists without evidence of other systemic metastases, it is termed a *solitary* metastasis. When the brain lesion occurs in the setting of other metastatic disease, it is called a *single* metastasis. The distinction is clinically significant, as the approach to treatment of a lone brain metastasis may differ from that of multiple lesions, or those that occur in the setting of advanced systemic disease. Single or solitary lesions (in some instances in patients with more than one brain metastasis [29]) may be appropriate for focal therapy with radiation (stereotactic radiosurgery) or surgery. Breast, colorectal and renal cell cancers are more likely to generate single lesions, while lung cancer and melanoma are more likely to cause multiple metastases [30]. When only one intracranial lesion is found, even if the patient is known to have cancer, there is a danger of misdiagnosis. In one study, 11% of patients with cancer and an isolated parenchymal lesion were found to have either a primary glioma or abscess, rather than metastatic disease [31].

Incidence of Brain Metastases in Children

Brain metastases are a rare complication in children and therefore the incidence is even more difficult to quantify. Vannucci and Baten conducted an analysis of autopsy data from 1951 through 1972 at Memorial Sloan-Kettering Cancer Center. Thirteen of 217 brains examined demonstrated tumor deposits; the authors projected the incidence of brain metastases in children with malignant tumors to be approximately 6% [32]. In this series, all patients with brain lesions had evidence of pulmonary disease arguing in favor of a hematogenous route of dissemination. Graus and colleagues conducted a retrospective review of brain metastases in children with solid tumors at the same institution from 1973–1982. They examined 139 post-mortem specimens and determined 18 patients had secondary tumors (12.9%) suggesting that the incidence had increased over time [33]. The brain lesions were found to be clinically symptomatic in 25 of the 31 patients. Sarcoma and germ cell tumors accounted for the most common systemic cancer to metastasize to the brain. Notably decreased was the number of brain metastases from Wilms tumor which represented 5% of diagnoses in this study and 13% in the previous study. In another report from France, Bouffet et al found 12 brain metastases out of 486 patients with solid tumors [34]. Osteogenic sarcoma, neuroblastoma, and Ewing's sarcoma each accounted for three incidents of brain metastasis. In all these studies, patients with brain lesions originating in the skull or dura were not included.

Pathophysiology

Metastasis is a dynamic process that involves multiple complex steps (Fig. 1). The specific mechanisms and sequence of events that lead to brain metastases are not yet fully understood. Both the cancer cell that metastasizes to the brain and the environment of the brain itself play important roles.

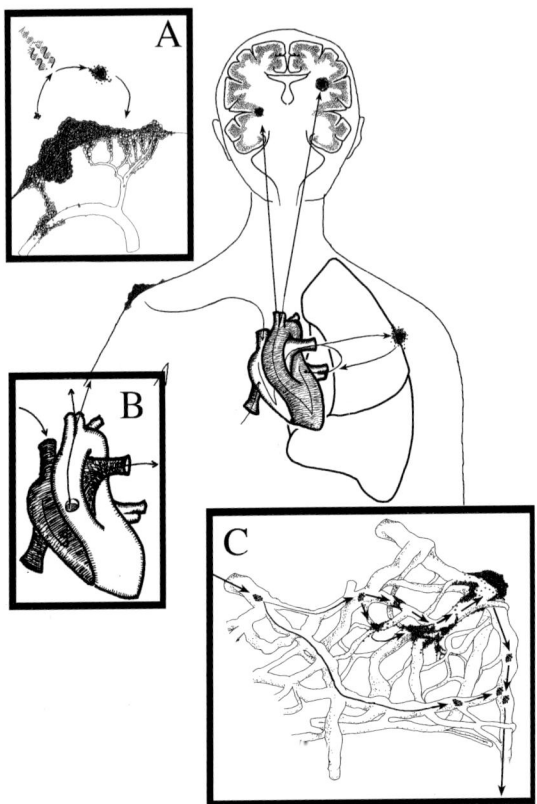

Figure 1. Pathophysiology of brain metastases. (A) A normal cell (1) undergoes multiple genetic mutations or epigenetic changes (2) to become a cancer (a melanoma as shown here). (3) It then proliferates uncontrollably and develops its own feeding vessels. (4) Angiogenesis invades the normal tissue stroma (5) and enters blood vessels or lymph channels (6). (B) The tumor gains access to the right side of the heart via the venous circulation (7). Cancer cells may be shunted to the left side of the heart via a patent foramen ovale or septal defect (8), or (C) more commonly, the cancer cells leave the heart via the pulmonary artery to reach the long capillary bed (9), where they may either form a metastasis (9) or pass through the capillary bed to reach the left atrium (10) from which tumor cells reach arterial circulation and seed the brain, usually at the gray matter/white matter junction. If the "soil" (brain) is hospitable, the tumor may leave brain capillaries and become a metastasis (11). From [18] with permission.

The Metastatic Cell

Most cancers arise from a single cell line and are therefore clonal. One hypothesis is that cancers arise from stem cells that are capable of self renewal, self-regulation and the ability to reconstitute all functional elements within their cell lineage [35]. Transformation of a stem cell leads to a cancer stem cell and these cells are believed to be relatively resistant to treatment and, thus, responsible for recurrence of tumor after initial response. As the cancer grows, daughter cells accumulate mutations that cause genetic instability and heterogeneity. It is believed that only about 15% of cells in a given tumor are capable of metastasis [36]; when a cell acquires this capacity has been debated. One premise is that the genetic changes necessary to confer invasive ability are present early in the course of disease. Another viewpoint is that a subpopulation of cells evolves during the progression of cancer, through acquisition of gene mutations and loss of tumor suppressors. Both hypotheses may be correct, and may in part account for why the timing of metastases differs among tumors. When tumor cells metastasize early, it is believed that a large number of cells have acquired the ability to do so. When metastases occur later in the course of disease, a much smaller proportion of cells may have developed these properties at a much later time [37].

In order for metastatic cells to desert the primary tumor, it must acquire a phenotype that allows it to detach, circulate and invade. Most carcinomas are composed of epithelial cells that demonstrate polarity, uniformity, and cohesiveness, allowing them to form well-organized structures. However, these qualities make them poorly suited to mobilize and invade other tissues. Mesenchymal cells, on the other hand, lack polarity, are highly variegated and are unrestricted by tight cell-to-cell adhesions. They are thereby better designed for migration [38]. During embryogenesis, cells are temporarily able to undergo a transformation from epithelial to mesenchymal cell. This *epithelial-mesenchymal transition* (EMT) occurs during gastrulation and organ formation, when cells are motile. It is also thought to be an essential part of tissue remodeling and wound healing [39]. The central event in EMT involves the loss of cell adhesion and detachment, which ultimately results in mobility of the cell. Tumor cells may be able to recover EMT and exploit it to facilitate their migration from the primary organ to a distant site. Multiple factors are thought to catalyze and support this metamorphosis. Recently, the activation of the phosphatidylinositol 3 kinase (PI3K)/ AKT pathway is proving to be one of the chief determinants of EMT induction [40].

The Microenvironment

Once the metastatic cell escapes from the primary tumor, what determines to where it will travel? Trafficking of most tumor cells occurs through the vascular or lymphatic system. From this, one might conclude that metastases would distribute in the pattern of blood or lymphatic flow from the primary cancer. This *mechanical* or *hemodynamic hypothesis of metastasis* was championed by James Ewing [41]. Most tumor cells ferry through vessels or lymphatics and many mechanically arrest in the first capillary or lymph-node bed they encounter. They may then establish a satellite tumor at this location. For example, colon cancers spread via the portal circulation to the liver; in breast cancer, the usual site of first metastasis is the axillary lymph nodes.

However, this mechanism does not account for all metastatic phenomena. Although muscle, kidney and skin are all highly vascular structures, they are rarely sites of metastases [2][42]. In 1889, Stephen Paget analyzed the autopsy results from 735 cases of breast cancer and observed that although the blood supply to the kidney and spleen was more generous, the liver was a more common organ for metastases [43]. He could not account for this finding by the random dispersion of metastatic cells, or by hemodynamics alone. He suggested there may be properties of the host organ itself that influence where tumor cells will eventually choose to settle. This led him to propose the "seed and soil" hypothesis [42]. He posited, "that the distribution of the secondary growth is not a matter of chance…when a plant goes to seed, its seeds are carried in all directions; but they can only live and grow if they fall on congenial soil." That is to say, the tumor cell (seed) can only flourish if it encounters a hospitable organ (soil).

Abundant evidence supports the "seed and soil", or *molecular recognition hypothesis*. As noted earlier, melanoma although infrequent, commonly metastases to the brain, but prostate cancer rarely does. Presumably, the "soil" of the brain is favorable for the melanoma "seeds". B16 melanoma cells in mice can be engineered to select specific organs (including the brain) for growth when the tumor cells are injected intravenously [44]. Tarin and colleagues studied patients with ovarian cancer who developed malignant ascites. They were treated with peritoneovenous shunts that drained fluid filled with tumor cells into the vena cava. Despite the fact that millions of these cells had free access to the circulation, metastatic disease rarely transpired, challenging the influence of the hemodynamic hypothesis [45].

These two theories are not mutually exclusive. Tumor cells reach other organs via vascular and lymphatic currents [46]. After they reach a particular organ, whether or not they succeed in establishing a satellite tumor depends on the suitability of the "soil". One study based on autopsy findings predicts the hemodynamic hypothesis may account for up to 66% of metastases, while 20% may be attributed to the molecular recognition hypothesis [47]. Local metastases may be accounted for by hemodynamic forces, while more distant spread may be attributed to molecular recognition between tumor cells and the host organ [48].

The "Metastatic Cascade"

A chain of elaborate and challenging steps, termed the "metastatic cascade" [49], must be completed for dissemination of cancer to occur. Not all the mechanisms and factors that drive this process have been identified, but an exhaustive list of growth factors, cytokines, immunologic mediators, and molecular pathways all play a role [50][49]. The sequence of events includes: detachment, intravasation, transport or embolization, extravasation, colonization, and angiogenesis (Table 2).

Table 2. Steps in the development of CNS metastases

Primary organ (e.g. breast cancer, melanoma)
Transformation
   Genetic change
   Growth
   Angiogenesis
   Invasion
Transportation
   Intravasation into blood or lymph vessel
   Circulation
   Arrest in 1st capillary bed

CNS organ (brain, spinal cord, leptomeninges)
Transportation
   Passage to arterial circulation
   Arrest in CNS capillary bed
   Extravasation
   Dormancy
   Angiogenesis and growth

From [18] with permission

Detachment

Once a normal cell acquires the genetic change(s) that transform it into a tumor cell, in order it metastasize, it must first disengage itself from the tumor mass. As in normal cells, tumor cell-to-cell adhesion is largely mediated by cadherins [51]. Cadherins are part of a larger group of cell surface proteins called cellular adhesion molecules (CAMs). CAMs are cell surface proteins that allow binding of cells to each other, or to the extracellular matrix (ECM). Of the different types of cadherins, epithelial cadherin (E-cadherin) is the pivotal protein involved in cell-cell interactions; it is essentially the "glue" that holds these cells together. Select tumor cells turn "off" E-cadherin, a critical event in detachment. In addition to loss of E-cadherin, the cells turn "on" neuronal cadherin (N-cadherin). N-cadherin promotes motility and invasion by allowing tumor cells to attach to and invade the underlying stroma [52]. Loss of adhesion is a vital step in EMT. Down-regulation of E-cadherin and up-regulation of N-cadherin are two key events that occur during EMT. Accordingly, cells with decreased expression of E-cadherin have a higher metastatic potential [51][53]. Some recent evidence suggests that the up-regulation of N-cadherin by itself may induce detachment and motility [54][55].

Intravasation

Once disassociated from the primary tumor, tumor cells destined for metastases move toward blood vessels [56]. They then breach the endothelial basement membrane and ECM. The ECM acts not only as a buttress for the overlying cells, but is also heavily involved in cell signaling, proliferation and coordinating migration.

The cells begin this process with the release of several factors to degrade the basement membrane. Matrix metalloproteins (MMPs) are one of the key proteolytic enzymes involved and are designed to degrade any number of proteins such as collagens, laminin and fibronectin. In non-neoplastic mitotically active cells, this allows remodeling of the ECM to accommodate progeny cells. MMPs have been classified according to their ability to degrade certain proteins. MMP-2 and MMP-9 are thought to be the most prominent in the development of metastases. They are classified as gelatinases because of their specific ability to degrade denatured collagen. Increased expression of MMP-9 has been found to be upregulated in both brain metastasis and primary brain tumors [57]. One study has found that all brain metastases examined expressed MMP-2; tumors that do not express MMP-2 are associated with improved survival [58]. MMPs express great diversity of function and may act at many other points along the metastatic cascade including cell proliferation, migration, differentiation, angiogenesis, and apoptosis. For example, they are one of the driving forces of EMT and they can also act to degrade E-cadherin [51]. Urokinase plasminogen activator (uPA) is another active protease. When bound to the cell surface molecule, urokinase plasminogen activator receptor (uPAR), activated uPA converts other zymogens into active proteases. The most notable of these is plasminogen, which is cleaved into plasmin. Plasmin can then activate other MMPs, especially types 1,2,3,9 and 14, or can directly digest fibrin. Accordingly, as with MMP-2, high levels of uPAR can signify a more aggressive course and a poor prognosis [59][49]. Aside from promoting the degradation of the basement membrane, both these proteases are also thought to activate growth factors and chemokines that ultimately encourage tumorigenesis [60].

Transport and Embolization

Cancer cells, like all other cells, depend on contact with the stromal elements in order to survive. Typically, once cells are within blood vessels and no longer anchored to their underlying matrix they undergo apoptosis, termed *anoikis*, Greek for "homelessness". Metastatic cells are resistant to anoikis. Over-expression of integrin-linked kinase (ILK), a protein implicated in the down-regulation of E-cadherin, is thought to contribute to resistance to anoikis [61]. More recently, a new anti-apoptotic molecule, TrkB, has also been identified. TrkB is a receptor for several protein growth factors that induce the survival and differentiation of cell populations [62]. The detached tumor cells must also withstand assault from natural killer cells, macrophages and other elements of the immune system [63] as well as endure mechanical destruction from velocity related shear forces. To overcome these forces, tumor cells often associate themselves with platelets and leukocytes which act as escorts. Selectins, another subset of CAMs belonging to leukocytes (L-selectin), platelets (P-selectin) and endothelial cells (E-selectin), allow tumor cells to attach to platelets and leukocytes, thus facilitating their transport. [64] This "piggy-back" method of travel results in microemboli that serve two purposes. It lends the individual tumor cells more bulk, thereby increasing the chances of successfully reaching and arresting in the capillary bed of the target organ [65]. It also provides a mantle of protection for the cells that may shield it from circulating macrophages and monocytes [64].

The formation of tumor microemboli is largely triggered by tissue factor (TF) expressed on the surface of malignant cells. TF is active in recruiting platelets and also initiating the clotting cascade. In one study, mice lacking platelets had a significantly lower chance to develop metastases from injected melanoma cells than did wild-type mice [66].

Most metastases reach the brain via blood vessels, i.e., hematogenous spread. After traveling through the venous circulation and passing through the heart, the errant tumor cell will settle in the first capillary bed it encounters, that of the lungs. From here, they follow the circulation to the left heart and then on to other organs. Roughly 20% of the cardiac output is shuttled to the brain; therefore, it is not surprising that tumors of the lung, either primary or secondary, are frequently the source of brain metastases. Spread through CSF does account for some instances of leptomeningeal propagation of tumor, and dural or parenchymal metastasis can result via direct extension from skull-based tumors [2].

Most brain metastases are found at the grey-white junction, where blood vessels narrow to a critical point to trap tumor emboli [30][67]. In addition, the distribution of cerebral blood flow is predominantly to the cerebral hemispheres (80%), then the cerebellum and brainstem. Accordingly, 85% of brain metastases are found in the cerebrum, 10–15% in the cerebellum and 3% in the brainstem [30]. These findings would appear to support the hemodynamic dissemination as the primary mechanism involved. However, for unknown reasons, gastrointestinal and pelvic tumors have an unusual propensity to travel to the posterior fossa; about 50% of single metastases from these tumors occur in the cerebellum [30][68]. This is most likely due to a molecular affinity between the tumor cells and this environment. Thus, in the brain, patterns of metastasis may adhere to both the hemodynamic and molecular recognition hypotheses.

In some cases, an area of tissue injury may present an attractive site for tumor cells to settle. This has been seen with metastases to the oral cavity, at the site of an extraction [69]. Nielsen and Posner describe a patient with adenocarcinoma of the cervix who developed brain metastases to an area of evolving infarction [70]. It may be that growth factors released after tissue injury play a role in galvanizing tumor proliferation at this site.

Different tumors may have different patterns of regional metastasis in the brain. Malignant melanoma prefers to plant in the grey matter rather than the grey-white junction. Infiltrating ductal carcinoma of the breast usually produces parenchymal metastases, while infiltrating lobular carcinoma is more likely to invade the leptomeninges [71].

Adhesion

Circulating tumor microemboli eventually arrest in a vascular bed, the process of arrest is related in part to tumor size, but also by binding of tumor cells to surface molecules on the endothelium called endothelial addressins. These molecules are unique to the capillaries of specific organs [72][73][74]. These proteins act as a berth for circulating tumor cells that express complementary proteins, such as integrins. Integrins, another subset of CAMs, are integral proteins embedded in the plasma membrane of cells. Their primary role is related to attachment of the cellular cytoskeleton to the ECM as well as signal transduction from the ECM to the cell. Some evidence suggests they are involved in adhesion of tumor cells to platelets during embolization, as well as induction of proteases such as MMPs during intravasation [65][75].

CD44 is another integral membrane protein that mediates tumor cell adhesion to the endothelium at the secondary site. Its protein expression is up-regulated in almost 50% of brain metastases, mostly in breast, thyroid and melanoma [76]. E-selectin expressed on endothelial cells may also aid in tumor cell adhesion [64].

Extravasation

This process, like intravasation, requires the degradation of the ECM. Accordingly, several of the same factors involved in intravasation, including MMPs and uPA, are also employed here. One of the more pivotal steps in extravasation involves the degradation of heparan sulfate proteoglycans (HSPG) in the basement membrane and ECM by heparinase endoglycosidase that digests HSPG chains. Normally expressed by platelets and leukocytes, heparinase may also be produced by other cells including astrocytes [77] and certain cancers such as prostate [50][78]. MMPs also aid in the dissolution of the basement membrane and activate growth factors that spur tumor growth. The uPA-uPAR complex is also active in restructuring the basement membrane and activating other proteases.

Tumor cells may gain access to the surrounding tissue by shear force. A small tumor focus, once lodged in a vessel, may begin to proliferate and grow to a critical mass that allows it to push through the endothelial cell layer of the blood vessel to contact the basement membrane.

Colonization

Once successfully invading tissue parenchyma, the cancer cells can now grow to form a mass. This is a crucial point in determining the fate of these itinerant cells. If they are not able to grow, they will remain arrested in a dormant state as a micrometastasis [79]. Micrometastases are defined as tumor foci less than or equal to 2 mm in greatest dimension. There may be countless numbers of these expectant cells scattered throughout the body, lying dormant until they attain the ability to proliferate. Some evidence suggests that the early steps of metastasis are relatively facile, and this last step of colonization is only rarely productive; therefore, it is considered the rate-limiting step of the cascade. One study describes that 80% of melanoma cells injected into mice survived to the point where they reach extravasation. However, less than 3% formed micrometastases, and only 1% continued on to form clinically apparent metastases [80].

The presence of these micrometastases may have substantial implications for prognosis. One study conducted by Braun and colleagues found that 36% of breast cancer patients with stage I, II or III disease demonstrated micrometastases in their bone marrow. Moreover, their presence was found to correlate with the risk of future relapse and death from disease [81].

Because they are clinically silent, these micrometastases may appear to be dormant. However, in all likelihood these clusters of cells are actively proliferating, but held in check by increased apoptosis and inhibition of angiogenesis. Thus, they will remain in this state until equipoise is disrupted and one or more cells has gained the ability for unrestrained growth [82].

Angiogenesis

All tissue, whether neoplastic or not, is dependent on an adequate blood supply. A tumor cannot grow beyond 1 to 2 mm^3 unless it acquires its own blood supply, usually via angiogenesis [83][84]. A number of factors that induce new blood vessels include vascular endothelial growth factor (VEGF), basic fibroblast growth factor (bFGF), platelet derived growth factor (PDGF), and epidermal growth factor (EGF) [82][85]; VEGF is probably the most significant. VEGF, also called vascular permeability factor (VPF), plays an important role in brain edema associated with tumors [86]. VEGF binds to its receptor on endothelial cells and induces neovascularization, increases permeability and activates uPA [87]. It may also be a surrogate marker for tumor growth and progression and may serve as a prognostic marker [87].

Angiogenesis is a multi-step process. First, the endothelial cells proliferate and penetrate the host ECM. They then assemble into vessels that are highly irregular compared with those of normal tissue. Migration and transformation of endothelial cells can be mediated by bFGF, which can also stimulate production of proteases [85]. These nascent vessels are malformed, of variable size, and haphazard in their orientation. They differ from their antecedent counterparts in that they lack the typical endothelial barrier. The endothelial cells are not as cohesive, and tight junctions are sparse. These factors conspire to make the new vasculature more permeable. The advantages of neovascularization are two-fold, for not only does it permit the tumor cells to flourish, but these more permeable vessels allow cells to easily enter the circulation, resulting in metastases [88].

Hypoxic ischemic factor (HIF) is another important mediator of angiogenesis. HIF-1 is closely related to tissue oxygenation. Under hypoxic cell conditions, as seen with metabolically overactive tumor cells, HIF-1 is up-regulated. This in turn triggers an up-regulation of other factors essential to improve oxygenation including

VEGF and erythropoietin [50]. The growth of dormant micrometastases may be suppressed by anti-angiogenesis factors released from the primary cancer. When the primary tumor is excised, these anti-angiogenesis mediators are removed resulting in precipitous growth of the distant metastases [82].

Cells of the surrounding stroma may also serve as pro-angiogenesis factors. These include indigenous endothelial cells that may secrete angiopoietin, which stimulates cell differentiation, as well as host macrophages that express multiple growth factors such as VEGF, TGF-β, and interleukin-8 [89][90].

Other Features Relevant to the Pathophysiology of Brain Metastases

The molecular processes governing the dissemination of cancer to the CNS are shared with those of other organ metastases. However, the brain has unique features including its microenvironment, the blood brain barrier (BBB), the absence of lymphatic drainage, and the lack of mitotically active neurons that combine to create a unique environment.

Biology of Brain Metastasis and the Microenvironment of the Brain

Brain metastases usually grow as well-circumscribed globoid lesions. On both gross and microscopic examinations, their borders appear distinct from the surrounding parenchyma, lending them to complete surgical excision. Microglial cells are the brain's macrophages, many of which are activated and form a clear boundary between the tumor mass and brain tissue [91], perhaps accounting for the usually well-circumscribed metastasis. The metastatic tumor is almost always associated with peritumoral vasogenic edema. The edema results in part from the leakage of protein and other substances across the disrupted BBB within the tumor. These substances, foreign to normal brain, diffuse from the tumor into the surrounding brain, thus increasing brain water. In addition, when VEGF is produced by the tumor, it may diffuse in the normal brain and increase permeability of normal vessels.

As discussed, primary tumors are composed of a heterogenous group of cells. By the time a subset of cells has arrived at a distant organ and established a metastasis, the biological behavior of this secondary lesion may differ greatly from that of the primary tumor [92]. Furthermore, the metastasis itself may be heterogeneous and two metastases within the brain may differ one from the other. These differences may in part explain why brain deposits do not respond to chemotherapy or radiation in the same way as the primary tumor, and why two metastases within the brain itself may differ in response. This heterogeneity presents a tremendous impediment to designing effective cancer therapeutics.

Blood Brain Barrier (BBB)

The BBB is composed of non-fenestrated, tightly packed endothelial cells that are closely associated with astrocyte foot processes. The barrier excludes most water-soluble chemotherapeutic agents given in standard doses, thus allowing the brain to serve as a sanctuary for micrometastases too small to disrupt the barrier. Eliminating sanctuary for tumor cells was the rationale for prophylactic CNS treatment of patients with leukemia and for prophylactic brain irradiation in patients with small-cell lung cancer [93]. It is not uncommon for patients with presumably cured cancer to develop solitary metastases in the brain years later. Breast cancer and melanoma in particular are the most common offenders [18].

CNS Lymphatics

Although it is generally recognized that the parenchyma of the brain and spinal cord do not possess lymphatic channels, the central nervous system (CNS) is not devoid of lymphatics [94][95]. Lymph channels along cranial nerves, particularly the olfactory nerve [96] and spinal nerves, are believed to drain materials from subarachnoid space (derived from brain interstitial fluid) into lymphatic system, especially cervical lymph nodes [97] [98]. Such drainage may account for cervical lymph node metastases from primary brain and leptomeningeal tumors [99] [100] [101] and may be a route by which the immune system recognizes nervous system antigens [96]. CNS lymphatics probably play no role in metastasis of extracranial tumors to brain.

References

1. Cappuzzo F, Mazzoni F, Maestri A, et al: Medical treatment of brain metastases from solid tumours. Forum (Genova) 2000; 10(2):137–148.
2. Posner JB: Neurologic Complications of Cancer. Philadelphia, F.A. Davis, 1995.
3. Lassman AB, DeAngelis LM: Brain metastases. Neurol Clin 2003; 21(1): 1–23.
4. Guomundsson KR: A survey of tumours of the central nervous system in Iceland during the 10-year period 1954–1963. Acta Neurologica Scandinavica 1970; 46:538–552.
5. Percy AK, Elveback LR, Okazaki H, et al: Neoplasms of the central nervous system. Epidemiologic considerations. Neurology 1972; 22:40–48.
6. Fogelholm R, Uutela T, Murros K: Epidemiology of central nervous system neoplasms. A regional survey in Central Finland. Acta Neurologica Scandinavica 1984; 69:129–136.

7. Walker AE, Robins M, Weinfeld FD: Epidemiology of brain tumors: The national survey of intracranial neoplasms. Neurology 1985; 35:219–226.

8. Posner JB, Chernik NL: Intracranial metastases from systemic cancer. Adv Neurol 1978; 19:575–587.

9. Cairncross JG, Kim J-H, Posner JB: Radiation therapy of brain metastases. Ann Neurol 1980; 7:529–541.

10. Pickren JW, Lopez G, Tsukada Y, et al: Brain metastases: An autopsy study. Cancer Treat Symp 1983; 2:295–313.

11. Shojania KG, Burton EC, McDonald KM, et al: Changes in rates of autopsy-detected diagnostic errors over time: a systematic review. JAMA 2003; 289(21):2849–2856.

12. Tham YL, Sexton K, Kramer R, et al: Primary breast cancer phenotypes associated with propensity for central nervous system metastases. Cancer 2006; 107(4):696–704.

13. Davis FG, McCarthy B, Jukich P: The descriptive epidemiology of brain tumors. Neuroimaging Clin N Am 1999; 9(4):581–594.

14. Johnson JD, Young B: Demographics of brain metastasis. Neurosurg Clin N Am 1996; 7(3):337–344.

15. Fogarty GB, Tartaguia C: The utility of magnetic resonance imaging in the detection of brain metastases in the staging of cutaneous melanoma. Clin Oncol (R Coll Radiol) 2006; 18(4):360–362.

16. Seute T, Leffers P, Wilmink JT, et al: Response of asymptomatic brain metastases from small-cell lung cancer to systemic first-line chemotherapy. J Clin Oncol 2006; 24(13):2079–2083.

17. Larcos G, Maisey MN: FDG-PET screening for cerebral metastases in patients with suspected malignancy. Nucl Med Commun 1996; 17(3):197–198.

18. Gavrilovic IT, Posner JB: Brain metastases: epidemiology and pathophysiology. J Neurooncol 2005; 75(1):5–14.

19. Barnholtz-Sloan JS, Sloan AE, Lai P, et al: Incidence proportions of brain metastases in patients diagnosed (1973 to 2001) in the metropolitan Detroit cancer surveillance system. J Clin Oncol 2004; 22(14):2865–2872.

20. Walker AE, Adamkiewitcz JJ: Pseudotumor cerebri associated with prolonged corticosteroid therapy: reports of four cases. JAMA 1964; 188:779–784.

21. Schouten LJ, Rutten J, Huveneers HAM, et al: Incidence of brain metastases in a cohort of patients with carcinoma of the breast, colon, kidney, and lung and melanoma. Cancer 2002; 94(10):2698–2705.

22. Madajewicz S, Karakousis C, West CR, et al: Malignant melanoma brain metastases. Review of Roswell Park Memorial Institute experience. Cancer 1984; 53(11):2550–2552.

23. Hutter A, Schwetye KE, Bierhals AJ, et al: Brain neoplasms: epidemiology, diagnosis, and prospects for cost-effective imaging. Neuroimaging Clin N Am 2003; 13(2):237–242.

24. Nussbaum ES, Djalilian HR, Cho KH, et al: Brain metastases - Histology, multiplicity, surgery, and survival. Cancer 1996; 78(8):1781–1788.
25. Bartelt S, Lutterbach J: Brain metastases in patients with cancer of unknown primary. J Neurooncol 2003; 64(3):249–253.
26. Polyzoidis KS, Miliaras G, Pavlidis N: Brain metastasis of unknown primary: a diagnostic and therapeutic dilemma. Cancer Treat Rev 2005; 31(4):247–255.
27. Gabos Z, Sinha R, Hanson J, et al: Prognostic significance of human epidermal growth factor receptor positivity for the development of brain metastasis after newly diagnosed breast cancer. J Clin Oncol 2006; 20;24(36):5658–63.
28. Daryanani D, Plukker JT, de Jong MA, et al: Increased incidence of brain metastases in cutaneous head and neck melanoma. Melanoma Res 2005; 15(2):119–124.
29. Nishizaki T, Saito K, Jimi Y, et al: The role of cyberknife radio-surgery/radiotherapy for brain metastases of multiple or large-size tumors. Minim Invasive Neurosurg 2006; 49(4):203–209.
30. Delattre J-Y, Krol G, Thaler HT, et al: Distribution of brain metastases. Arch Neurol 1988; 45:741–744.
31. Patchell RA, Tibbs PA, Walsh JW: A randomized trial of surgery in the treatment of single metastases to the brain. N Engl J Med 1990; 322: 494–500.
32. Vannucci RC, Baten M: Cerebral metastatic disease in childhood. Neurology 1974; 24(10):981–985.
33. Graus F, Walker RW, Allen JC: Brain metastases in children. J Pediatr 1983; 103(4):558–561.
34. Bouffet E, Doumi N, Thiesse P, et al: Brain metastases in children with solid tumors. Cancer 1997; 79(2):403–410.
35. Schulenburg A, Ulrich-Pur H, Thurnher D, et al: Neoplastic stem cells: A novel therapeutic target in clinical oncology. Cancer 2006; 107(10):2512–2520.
36. Fidler IJ, Kripke ML: Metastasis results from preexisting variant cells within a malignant tumor. Science 1977; 197(4306):893–895.
37. Pantel K, Brakenhoff RH: Dissecting the metastatic cascade. Nat Rev Cancer 2004; 4(6):448–456.
38. Lee JM, Dedhar S, Kalluri R, et al: The epithelial-mesenchymal transition: new insights in signaling, development, and disease. J Cell Biol 2006; 172(7): 973–981.
39. Hay ED: The mesenchymal cell, its role in the embryo, and the remarkable signaling mechanisms that create it. Dev Dyn 2005; 233(3):706–720.
40. Larue L, Bellacosa A: Epithelial-mesenchymal transition in development and cancer: role of phosphatidylinositol 3' kinase/AKT pathways. Oncogene 2005; 24(50):7443–7454.
41. Ewing J: Metastasis. In: Ewing J, (ed): Neoplastic Diseases: A Treatise on Tumours. Philadelphia, W.B. Saunders, 1940:62–74.

42. Fidler IJ, Yano S, Zhang RD, et al: The seed and soil hypothesis: vascularisation and brain metastases. Lancet Oncol 2002; 3(1):53–57.

43. Paget S: The distribution of secondary growths in cancer of the breast. Cancer Metastasis Rev. 1989; 8(2):98–101.

44. Fidler IJ: The pathogenesis of cancer metastasis: the 'seed and soil' hypothesis revisited. Nat Rev Cancer 2003; 3(6):453–458.

45. Tarin D, Price JE, Kettlewell MG, et al: Mechanisms of human tumor metastasis studied in patients with peritoneovenous shunts. Cancer Res 1984; 44(8):3584–3592.

46. Chambers AF, MacDonald IC, Schmidt EE, et al: Steps in tumor metastasis: New concepts from intravital videomicroscopy. Cancer Metastasis Rev 1995; 14(4):279–301.

47. Weiss L: Comments on hematogenous metastatic patterns in humans as revealed by autopsy. Clin Exp Metastasis 1992; 10:191–199.

48. Sugarbaker EV: Cancer metastasis: a product of tumor-host interactions. Curr Probl Cancer 1979; 3(7):1–59.

49. Nathoo N, Chahlavi A, Barnett GH, et al: Pathobiology of brain metastases. J Clin Pathol 2005; 58(3):237–242.

50. Puduvalli VK: Brain metastases: biology and the role of the brain microenvironment Curr Oncol Rep 2001; 3(6):467–475.

51. Cavallaro U, Christofori G: Cell adhesion in tumor invasion and metastasis: loss of the glue is not enough. Biochim Biophys Acta Rev Cancer 2001; 1552(1).39–45.

52. Steeg PS: Tumor metastasis: mechanistic insights and clinical challenges. Nat Med 2006; 12(8):895–904.

53. Hirohashi S: Inactivation of the E-cadherin-mediated cell adhesion system in human cancers. Am J Pathol 1998;153(2):333–339.

54. Nieman MT, Prudoff RS, Johnson KR, et al: N-cadherin promotes motility in human breast cancer cells regardless of their E-cadherin expression. J Cell Biol 1999; 147(3):631–644.

55. Li G, Satyamoorthy K, Herlyn M: N-cadherin-mediated intercellular interactions promote survival and migration of melanoma cells. Cancer Res 2001; 61(9):3819–3825.

56. Wyckoff JB, Jones JG, Condeelis JS, et al: A critical step in metastasis: *In vivo* analysis of intravasation at the primary tumor. Cancer Research 2000; 60(9):2504–2511.

57. Arnold SM, Young AB, Munn RK, et al: Expression of p53, bcl-2, E-cadherin, matrix metalloproteinase-9, and tissue inhibitor of metalloproteinases-1 in paired primary tumors and brain metastasis. Clin Cancer Res 1999; 5(12):4028–4033.

58. Jäälinojä J, Herva R, Korpela M, et al: Matrix metalloproteinase 2 (MMP-2) immunoreactive protein is associated with poor grade and survival in brain neoplasms. J Neurooncol 2000; 46(1):81–90.

59. Boyd TS, Mehta MP: Radiosurgery for brain metastases. Neurosurg Clin N Am 1999; 10(2):337–350.
60. Folgueras AR, Pendas AM, Sanchez LM, et al: Matrix metalloproteinases in cancer: from new functions to improved inhibition strategies. Int J Dev Biol 2004; 48(5–6):411–424.
61. Attwell S, Roskelley C, Dedhar S: The integrin-linked kinase (ILK) suppresses anoikis. Oncogene 2000; 19(33):3811–3815.
62. Douma S, Van LT, Zevenhoven J, et al: Suppression of anoikis and induction of metastasis by the neurotrophic receptor TrkB. Nature 2004; 430(7003):1034–1039.
63. Hanna N: Inhibition of experimental tumor metastasis by selective activation of natural killer cells. Cancer Res 1982; 42(4):1337–1342.
64. Borsig L, Wong R, Hynes RO, et al: Synergistic effects of L- and P-selectin in facilitating tumor metastasis can involve non-mucin ligands and implicate leukocytes as enhancers of metastasis. Proc Natl Acad Sci U S A 2002; 99(4):2193–2198.
65. Felding-Habermann B, O'Toole TE, et al: Integrin activation controls metastasis in human breast cancer. Proc Natl Acad Sci USA 2001; 98(4):1853–1858.
66. Camerer E, Qazi AA, Duong DN, et al: Platelets, protease-activated receptors, and fibrinogen in hematogenous metastasis. Blood 2004; 104(2):397–401.
67. Hwang TL, Close TP, Grego JM, et al: Predilection of brain metastasis in gray and white matter junction and vascular border zones. Cancer 1996; 77(8):1551–1555.
68. Cascino TL, Leavengood JM, Kemeny N, et al: Brain metastases from colon cancer. J Neurooncol 1983; 1:203–209.
69. Hirshberg A, Leibovich P, Horowitz I, et al: Metastatic tumors to postextraction sites. J Oral Maxillofac Surg 1993; 51(12):1334–1337.
70. Nielson SL, Posner JB: Brain metastasis localized to an area of infarction. J Neurooncol 1983; 1:191–195.
71. Smith DB, Howell A, Harris M, et al: Carcinomatous meningitis associated with infiltrating lobular carcinoma of the breast. Eur J Surg Oncol 1985; 11:33–36.
72. Pasqualini R, Arap W: Profiling the molecular diversity of blood vessels. Cold Spring Harb Symp Quant Biol 2002; 67:223–225.
73. Trepel M, Arap W, Pasqualini R: In vivo phage display and vascular heterogeneity: implications for targeted medicine. Curr Opin Chem Biol 2002; 6(3):399–404.
74. Brayton J, Qing Z, Hart MN, et al: Influence of adhesion molecule expression by human brain microvessel endothelium on cancer cell adhesion. J Neuroimmunol 1998; 89(1–2):104–112.
75. Friedl P, Wolf K: Tumour-cell invasion and migration: diversity and escape mechanisms. Nat Rev Cancer 2003; 3(5):362–374.

76. Harabin-Slowinska M, Slowinski J, Konecki J, et al: Expression of adhesion molecule CD44 in metastatic brain tumors. Folia Neuropathol 1998; 36(3):179–184.
77. Marchetti D, Li J, Shen R: Astrocytes contribute to the brain-metastatic specificity of melanoma cells by producing heparanase. Cancer Res 2000; 60(17):4767–4770.
78. Kosir MA, Wang W, Zukowski KL, et al: Degradation of basement membrane by prostate tumor heparanase. J Surg Res 1999; 81(1):42–47.
79. Hedley BD, Allan AL, Chambers AF: Tumor dormancy and the role of metastasis suppressor genes in regulating ectopic growth. Future Oncol 2006; 2(5):627–641.
80. Luzzi KJ, MacDonald IC, Schmidt EE, et al: Multistep nature of metastatic inefficiency - Dormancy of solitary cells after successful extravasation and limited survival of early micrometastases. Am J Pathol 1998; 153(3): 865–873.
81. Braun S, Pantel K, Muller P, et al: Cytokeratin-positive cells in the bone marrow and survival of patients with stage I, II, or III breast cancer. N Engl J Med 2000; 342(8):525–533.
82. Kirsch M, Schackert G, Blkack PM: Angiogenesis, metastasis, and endogenous inhibition. J Neuro-Oncol 2000; 50(1–2):173–180.
83. Folkman J: Tumor angiogenesis: therapeutic implications. N Engl J Med 1971; 285(21):1182–1186.
84. Folkman J: How is blood vessel growth regulated in normal and neoplastic tissue? G.H.A. Clower Memorial Award Lecture. Cancer Res 1986; 46: 467–473.
85. Folkman J, Klagsbrun M: Angiogenic factors. Science 1987; 235(4787): 442–447.
86. Machein MR, Plate KH: VEGF in brain tumors. J Neurooncol 2000; 50(1–2): 109–120.
87. Poon RT, Fan ST, Wong J: Clinical implications of circulating angiogenic factors in cancer patients. J Clin Oncol 2001; 19(4):1207–1225.
88. McDonald DM, Baluk P: Significance of blood vessel leakiness in cancer. Cancer Res 2002; 62(18):5381–5385.
89. Bergers G, Benjamin LE: Tumorigenesis and the angiogenic switch. Nat Rev Cancer 2003; 3(6):401–410.
90. Joyce JA: Therapeutic targeting of the tumor microenvironment. Cancer Cell 2005; 7(6):513–520.
91. He BP, Wang JJ, Zhang X, et al: Differential reactions of microglia to brain metastasis of lung cancer. Mol Med 2006; 12(7–8):161–170.
92. Klein CA, Blankenstein TJ, Schmidt-Kittler O, et al: Genetic heterogeneity of single disseminated tumour cells in minimal residual cancer. Lancet 2002; 360(9334):683–689.

93. Auperin A, Arriagada R, Pignon JP, et al: Prophylactic cranial irradiation for patients with small-cell lung cancer in complete remission. Prophylactic Cranial Irradiation Overview Collaborative Group. N Engl J Med 1999; 341(7):476–484.
94. Foldi M: The brain and the lymphatic system (I). Lymphology 1996; 29(1): 1–9.
95. Foldi M: The brain and the lymphatic system (II). Lymphology 1996; 29(1):10–14.
96. Knopf PM, Cserr HF, Nolan SC, et al: Physiology and immunology of lymphatic drainage of interstitial and cerebrospinal fluid from the brain. Neuropathol Appl Neurobiol 1995; 21:175–180.
97. Johnston M, Zakharov A, Papaiconomou C, et al: Evidence of connections between cerebrospinal fluid and nasal lymphatic vessels in humans, non-human primates and other mammalian species. Cerebrospinal Fluid Res 2004: 1(1):2.
98. Koh L, Zakharov A, Johnston M: Integration of the subarachnoid space and lymphatics: is it time to embrace a new concept of cerebrospinal fluid absorption? Cerebrospinal Fluid Res 2005; 20, 2:6.
99. Moon KS, Jung S, Lee MC, et al: Metastatic glioblastoma in cervical lymph node after repeated craniotomies: report of a case with diagnosis by fine needle aspiration. J Korean Med Sci 2004; 19(6):911–914.
100. Brown MT, McClendon RE, Gockerman JP: Primary central nervous system lymphoma with systemic metastasis: case report and review. J Neurooncol 1995; 23(3):207–221.
101. Barone TA, Plunkett RJ, Hohmann P, et al: An experimental model of human leukemic meningitis in the nude rat. Blood 1997; 90(1):298–305.

the patients in this study and it also cost less than radiosurgery. Given the fact that the cost difference between HSRT and radiosurgery ($4,119) reported in this study is relatively large, it is worth considering HSRT as a less costly treatment for brain metastases. Based on the findings reported here, HSRT could play a role in reducing the costs of treating brain metastases if its advantages could be more definitively demonstrated clinically.

However, the interpretation of the studies discussed above from the neuro-surgeon's perspective differs. The two studies were funded primarily by manufac-turers of radiosurgical equipment and were viewed with caution by one neurosurgeon in 1995.[7] He noted that the authors strongly advocate the use of radiosurgery in the treatment of brain metastases, as well as several types of benign and malignant intracranial tumors. He also acknowledged that adequate cost and outcome data exist to support the authors' claim that radiosurgery is a preferable treatment for brain metastases. Dr. Ciric believes that the authors give the impression that radiosurgery is unquestionably more cost effective than surgical resection or whole brain radiation, while resulting in similar outcomes.[7]

However, Dr. Ciric points out that the results presented above should be inter-preted with more caution than the authors imply. He raises several concerns that may have influenced the strong conclusions presented in these studies. First, he explains that the authors may have been biased since they received funding from radiosurgical manufacturers. Second, he believes that more complete cost infor-mation could have been reported such as the length and cost of hospital stays for patients who underwent noncomplicated surgical resection and total treatment cost and the side effects of surgical resection versus radiosurgery. He makes the point that even if the procedure itself is more cost effective, we must consider associated costs relating to follow-up and rehabilitation as well. Third, Dr. Ciric takes issue with the authors' claim that a reduction in the annual volume of radiosurgery proce-dures by almost 40% would result in equal incremental cost effectiveness between radiosurgery and surgical resection. However, he astutely points out that the authors ignore the fact that superior cost effectiveness of radiosurgery could result in an increase in the number of total procedures performed, driving up the total cost of treatment overall for society.[7]

Recommendations for Future Research

Since the above studies were published in the mid-1990s, radiosurgery with the Leskell Gamma Knife®, manufactured by Elekta, has become the standard of care for many brain tumors, including brain metastases. Elekta reports that approxi-mately 300,000 patients have received Gamma Knife® radiosurgery to date, with about 35,000 patients receiving the treatment annually.[8] In 2006, American Shared Hospital Services reported that the Gamma Knife unit costs approximately $2.9 million, with reimbursement ranging from $7,500 to $9,500 per procedure on a usage-only basis.[9] Currently, there are over 100 Gamma Knife centers in the United States and over 200 Gamma Knife units have been installed worldwide.[9] In early 2006, the Centers for Medicaid and Medicare Services announced changes to its reimbursement policies that established payment coding for the Gamma Knife procedure.[10] These changes formally acknowledged Gamma Knife therapy as the standard of care in radiosurgery and increased reimbursement payment for Gamma Knife procedures by 28 percent.[10]

While these changes signal the emergence of the Gamma Knife as the standard of care for brain metastases, unanswered questions about the economics of this therapy still remain. There is a lack of published information available on the per-patient and societal costs of this therapy specifically for patients with brain metastases. Little is known about the cost-effectiveness, out-of-pocket costs, and the costs of potential side effects associated with the procedure. It is also important to consider the costs of clinical complications resulting from extended hospital stays as well as costs associated with absence from work and normal activity. Rigorous economic analyses including cost data for Gamma Knife radiosurgery are needed in order to adequately assess the economic impact of this therapy. As the number of Gamma Knife procedures increases, the opportunity to systematically collect and analyze cost data on patients with brain metastases exists, but we cannot begin to explore cost-containment strategies until such data are collected and analyzed.

Acknowledgments

We thank Veena Shankaran MD and Motasem Alkhatib MD for helpful comments and critiques of earlier drafts of this manuscript.

References

1. Mehta M, Noyes W, Craig B, et al. A cost-effectiveness and cost-utility analysis of radiosurgery vs. resection for single-brain metastases. Int J Radiat Oncol Biol Phys 1997;39(2):445–54.
2. Noordijk EM, Vecht CJ, Haaxma-Reiche H, et al. The choice of treatment of single brain metastasis should be based on extracranial tumor activity and age. Int J Radiat Oncol Biol Phys 1994;29(4):711–7.
3. Patchell RA, Tibbs PA, Walsh JW, et al. A randomized trial of surgery in the treatment of single metastases to the brain. N Engl J Med 1990;322(8):494–500.
4. Auchter RM, Lamond JP, Alexander E, et al. A multiinstitutional outcome and prognostic factor analysis of radiosurgery for resectable single brain metastasis. Int J Radiat Oncol Biol Phys 1996;35(1):27–35.
5. Rutigliano MJ, Lunsford LD, Kondziolka D, Strauss MJ, Khanna V, Green M. The cost effectiveness of stereotactic radiosurgery versus surgical resection in

the treatment of solitary metastatic brain tumors. Neurosurgery 1995;37(3): 445–53; discussion 53–5.

6. Manning MA, Cardinale RM, Benedict SH, et al. Hypofractionated stereotactic radiotherapy as an alternative to radiosurgery for the treatment of patients with brain metastases. Int J Radiat Oncol Biol Phys 2000;47(3):603–8.

7. Ciric I. Comment on: The cost effectiveness of stereotactic radiosurgery versus surgical resection in the treatment of solitary metastatic brain tumors. Neuro-surgery 1995;37(3):453–5.

8. Gamma Knife Surgery. Elekta Website. http://www.elekta.com/healthcare_ international_gamma_knife_surgery.php Accessed February 15, 2007.

9. Gamma Knife. American Shared Hospital Services Website. http:// www.ashs.com/gammaknife.htm Accessed February 15, 2007.

10. Gamma Knife(R) Surgery Reimbursement for 2006 Solidifies Efficacy of Technology as Standard of Care in Radiosurgery. News Release January 12, 2006.   http://salesandmarketingnetwork.com/news_release.php?ID=2009472 Accessed February 15, 2007. . The Healthcare Sales and Marketing Network.

3. Neuroimaging of Parenchymal Brain Metastases

Matthew T. Walker, MD and Vipul Kapoor, MD

Introduction

Metastatic disease to the central nervous system (CNS) is common and accounts for approximately 37% of intracranial neoplasms [1]. Autopsy studies have shown that 24% of patients who die from cancer have intracranial metastasis and the estimated annual incidence is approximately 170,000 cases per year [2]. Earlier detection and improved treatment of primary malignancies have contributed to the increasingly important role of imaging to detect CNS dissemination.

Intracranial metastases occur in the brain parenchyma, leptomeningeal layer (arachnoid lining, subarachnoid space and pial surface) and pachymeningeal layer (dura). The majority of intracranial metastases are parenchymal and are frequently symptomatic. This chapter will focus on imaging detection of parenchymal metastasis.

Imaging plays a critical role in the initial diagnosis, treatment and follow-up of brain metastasis. At presentation, imaging is used to establish the presence or absence of brain metastasis and characterize important elements such as multiplicity (solitary versus multiple), location and secondary effects (mass effect). During and after treatment, imaging is used to help monitor therapeutic response and survey for recurrence. Magnetic resonance imaging is the imaging study of choice.

Epidemiology

In the US, approximately 170,000 cancer patients develop brain metastases annually, and 24% (11–35% in different series) of patients with deaths related to cancer have intracranial metastasis [1, 2]. The primary tumor determines the age of presentation of brain metastases, occurring most commonly between 35–70 years of age [3]. The most common adult primary tumors to metastasize to the brain, in decreasing order of frequency, are lung, breast, melanoma, renal and colon cancer [1, 4]. Gender predilection of brain metastases follows the primary tumor: lung cancer metastasis is most common in male patients and breast cancer is most common in female patients. The incidence of parenchymal brain metastases in women with hormone receptor negative breast cancer is particularly high [5]. Brain metastases in children are less frequent, with an incidence of approximately 5% and most common with neuroblastoma and sarcomas [6].

Presentation

Approximately 15% of patients will have intracranial metastatic disease at the time of their primary diagnosis. Patients with a primary diagnosis and neurological symptoms will have brain metastases 45% of the time [7]. The most common symptoms include headache, weakness and mental status change, and are primarily caused by local mass effect, brain inflammation and increased intracranial pressure. Focal neurological deficits occur and can often be explained by knowledge of functional neuroanatomy. Symptoms may have a gradual presentation, or may present acutely as a seizure or in a "stroke like" manner with hemorrhage into the lesion.

Pathophysiology and Imaging Correlates

Systemic tumors can spread by direct extension or via the hematogenous and lymphatic routes. Dissemination to the brain parenchyma is primarily arterial hematogenous although direct extension by skull, sinonasal or a nasopharyngeal tumor does occur. The brain is generally devoid of any significant lymphatic channels and does not contribute to parenchymal brain metastasis. Efferent lymphatics are present in many mammalian species at the level of the olfactory nerves and drain into the nasal cavity but are not a likely source of significant intracranial access [8].

The predominant route of access to the brain parenchyma for systemic tumors is via arterial hematogenous spread. The distribution of metastases tends to reflect the relative amount of blood flow to the brain: areas with higher volumes of flow (middle cerebral artery territory) tend to have a higher prevalence of metastatic foci. This phenomenon applies to any arterial embolic process including stroke and septic emboli. The higher flow anterior circulation accounts for approximately 80% of parenchymal metastases compared to 20% for the lower flow posterior circulation (15% cerebellum, 5% brainstem) [9]. The imaging correlate is a higher frequency of metastases to the frontal and parietal lobes and adjacent watershed areas compared to the temporal and occipital lobes.

Parenchymal metastatic lesions characteristically occur at the grey-white matter junction and watershed areas, which on a basic level directly relates to the typical size of the tumor emboli and the size of the penetrating cortical artery. As the penetrating artery extends from the cortex into the subcortical white matter there is a dramatic decrease in the diameter of the arterioles thus creating a convenient location for a tumor embolus to be deposited [10]. It is intuitive that tumor emboli in the 100–200 micron range will become lodged in the 50–150 micron arterioles as originally postulated by Watanabe in 1954 and recalled by Henson and Urich in 1982 [11].

After the parenchymal metastasis is established, a variety of reactions occur that reflect the underlying nature of the disease including neovascularization, reactive astrocytosis and microglial activation [12]. Actively growing tumor nodules require energy and quickly outstrip their ATP sources. In response to this demand, neovascularity occurs that provides increased access to ATP for continued growth. These blood vessels do not maintain the blood-brain-barrier and are leaky, which results in enhancement on post-contrast MRI. On perfusion imaging neovascularity is manifested as elevated cerebral blood volume [13, 14]. Reactive astrocytosis occurs within the brain parenchyma adjacent to metastatic lesions and contributes to the edema response around a lesion. Microglial activation occurs in the setting of tumor necrosis and contributes to abnormal parenchymal signal. Neovascularity and resultant vascular permeability, reactive astrocytosis and microglial activation all manifest as contributions to T2 hyperintensity around a parenchymal metastasis. Another characteristic to note is the presence of hemorrhage, which can be delineated as susceptibility effect on gradient echo imaging. Hemorrhage within a metastatic lesion is common (∼20%) and can be identified with certain MRI pulse sequences particularly the gradient recalled echo sequence (GRE) [15]. GRE is sensitive for the presence or absence of blood and, in an unknown case, can help focus the differential on those lesions that tend to bleed. Melanin can be detected on MRI and is characterized as T1 hyperintensity and T2 isointensity. When present, melanocytic tumors are implicated, typically melanoma.

Neuroimaging

Introduction

MRI is the imaging modality of choice in the clinical setting of suspected or known intracranial metastatic disease due to superior sensitivity and specificity, soft tissue contrast, spatial resolution, multiplanar localization and absence of beam hardening artifact in the posterior fossa and at the skull base. There are a few good reasons to not obtain an MRI in this clinical scenario including: (1) MRI safety contraindications such as pacemakers or cochlear implants, (2) claustrophobia not manageable with sedation or anesthesia (3) patient refusal and (4) lack of access to MRI for whatever reason. In a patient with a known gadolinium allergy it is

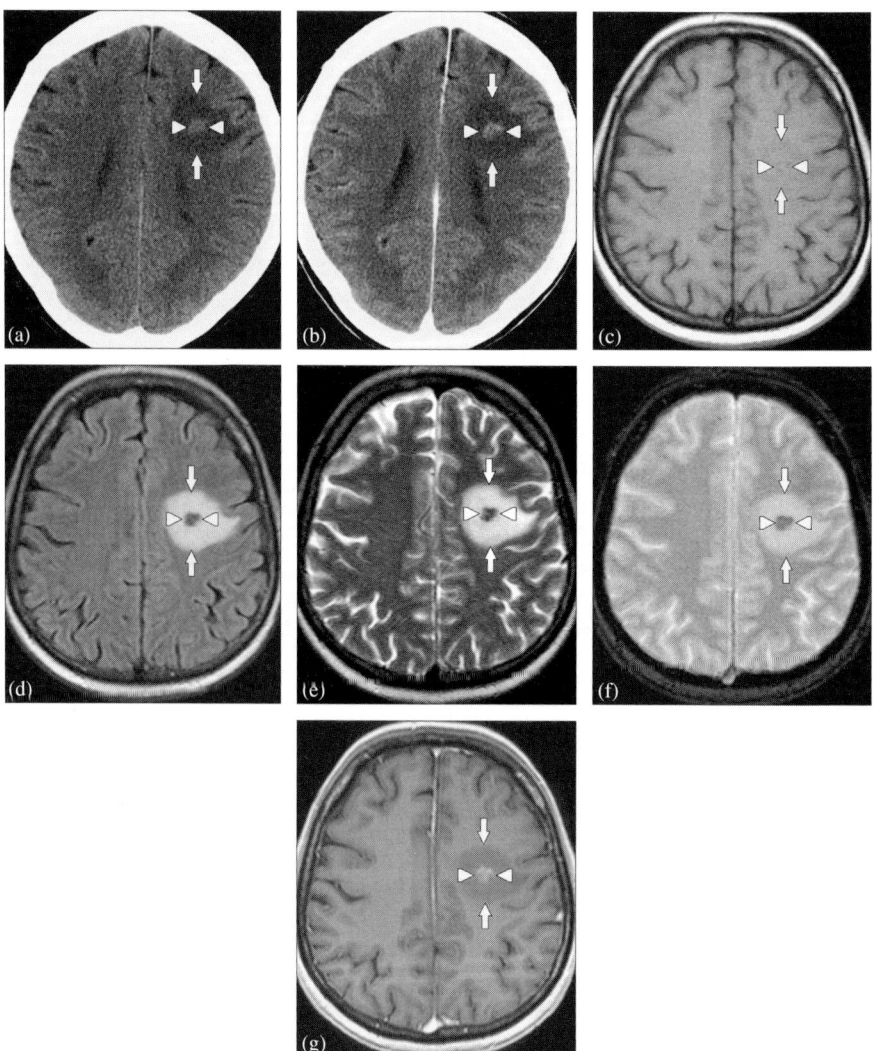

Figure 2. (a) **Hemorrhagic Choricarcinoma Metastasis**. Non-contrast axial CT scan superior to the ventricles shows a rounded hyperdense mass (arrowheads) with a rim of hypodensity (arrows) extending from the margins of the mass in the left frontal lobe. The mass is either hemorrhagic or highly cellular. (b) Contrast-enhanced axial CT scan shows subtle enhancement of the lesion (arrowheads), which will become more conspicuous on MR. The vasogenic edema (arrows) does not enhance. (c) Axial T1-weighted image shows heterogeneous signal in the mass (arrowheads) including subtle T1 shortening that represents blood products. The vasogenic edema (arrows) is subtle. (d) Axial FLAIR image highlights the vasogenic edema (arrows). The mass (arrow heads) is moderately hypointense suggestive of blood. (e) Axial T2-weighted image demonstrates hypointensity in the mass (arrowheads) indicative of blood products.

contemporary 1.5 Tesla MR systems can perform anatomical pulse sequences such as T1, T2, FLAIR, GRE, diffusion and post-contrast studies. More sophisticated systems can perform MR Perfusion, MR Spectroscopy and fiber tract analyses, which are not required but extremely helpful in certain clinical scenarios including unknown solitary lesions and treated lesions.

T1-Weighted Imaging

Routine T1-weighted pulse sequences use the spin-echo technique that renders parenchyma grey signal and free fluid black signal intensity. The majority of metastatic lesions are iso- to hypointense on T1 (Fig 1b) [18]. Intrinsic T1 hyperintensity "also know as T1-shortening" can be seen in three circumstances: (1) hemorrhage, (2) melanin, indicating and (3) necrosis with release of intracellular paramagnetic metals (copper, iron) and free radical peroxidation (Fig 2c) [19]. Calcification has a variable appearance and is often inconspicuous or hypointense.

T2/FLAIR Imaging

Routine T2-weighted sequences are either spin echo (SE) or fast spin echo (FSE) acquisitions: the latter has shorter image acquisition time but less chemical shift properties and less susceptibility effects (ability to detect hemorrhage), which may or may not be desirable depending upon the lesion [20]. SE and FSE T2 render CSF hyperintense and brain parenchyma relatively hypointense. FLAIR (fluid-attenuation inversion recovery) is a special T2-weighted sequence that suppresses fluid signal and renders CSF as hypointense (Figs 1c, 2d). This results in excellent T2 contrast in the parenchyma especially on the margins of the ventricles and cortex but it does not perform well in the posterior fossa [21]. The majority of metastatic lesions are hyperintense on T2-weighted imaging. If a metastatic lesion hemorrhages, the signal will vary depending upon the age of the bleed. In general, hemorrhage in a metastasis is T2 hypointense in the acute stage and T2 hyperintense in the subacute stage (Fig 2e) [22]. Hemorrhage should be confirmed on other sequences and if present the differential diagnosis can be narrowed. T2 hypointensity in a metastasis is not specific for hemorrhage: mucinous adenocarcinomas are characteristically T2-hypointense due to microcalcification and lymphoma is T2-hypointense due to high nuclear-to-cytoplasmic ratios (Figs 1d, 3b) [4]. Vasogenic edema in the brain parenchyma is T2 hyperintense.

Figure 2. The differential would include a mucinous metastasis due to micromineralization. The vasogenic edema (arrows) remains hyperintense. (f) Axial GRE sequence shows hypointense signal (arrowheads) defining the mass and indicating the presence of blood. There is no evidence for blood in the surrounding edema (arrows). (g) Axial T1-weighted (MPRAGE) post-gadolinium image improves conspicuity of the mass (arrowheads). The edema (arrows) does not enhance and is a reaction to the presence of a metastasis.

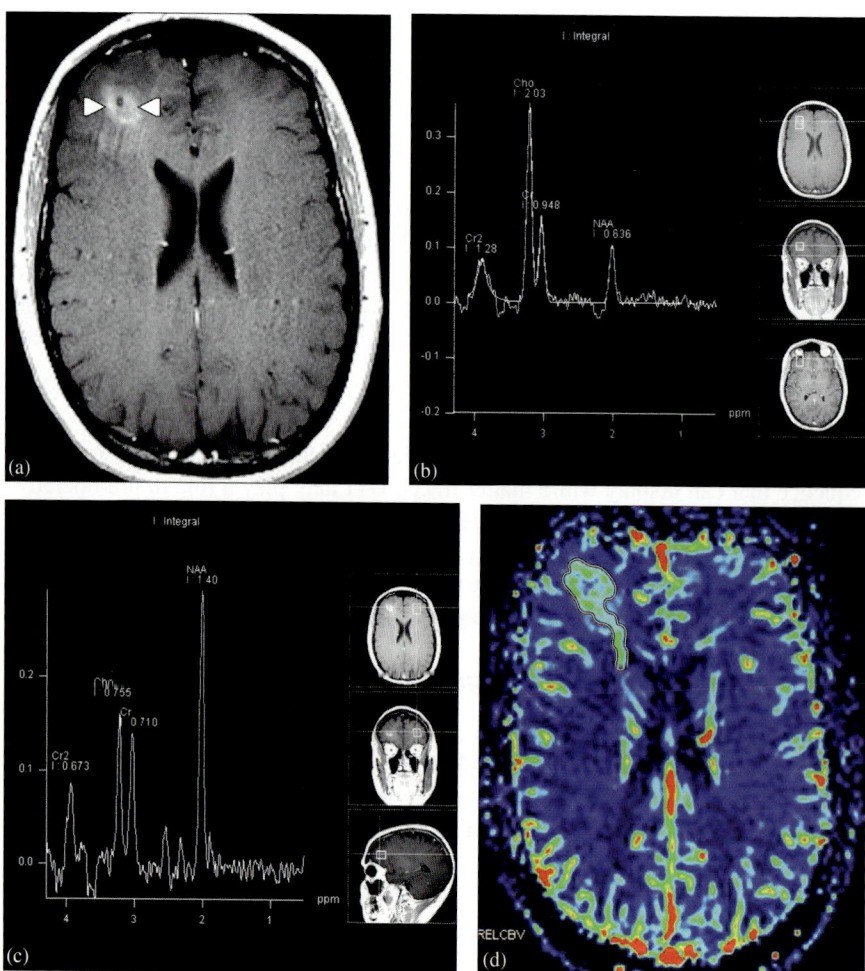

Figure 4. (a) **Lung Metastasis**. Axial T1-weighted (MPRAGE) post-gadolinium image shows an enhancing lesion (arrowheads) in the right frontal lobe. (b) MR Spectroscopy (single voxel, long TE = 144 ms) of the enhancing right frontal lesion demonstrates a classic tumor profile including elevated choline (Cho) relative to creatine (Cr) and n-acetyl aspartate (NAA). The Cho/Cr ratio is 2.1 and Cho/NAA ratio is 3.2, both compatible with tumor. A line connecting the Cho, Cr, and NAA peaks is called a reverse Hunter's angle, indicative of a tumor profile. (c) MR Spectroscopy (single voxel, long TE = 144 ms) of contralateral normal white matter in the same patient shows a normal spectral pattern. A line connecting Cho, Cr and NAA would create Hunter's angle, which is a normal profile. Compare to Figure 4b. (d) MR Perfusion (contrast-enhanced, echo-planar gradient echo technique) CBV parametric map identifies elevated CBV corresponding to the enhancing lesion. The rCBV ratio compared to contralateral white matter is 3:1, compatible with tumor.

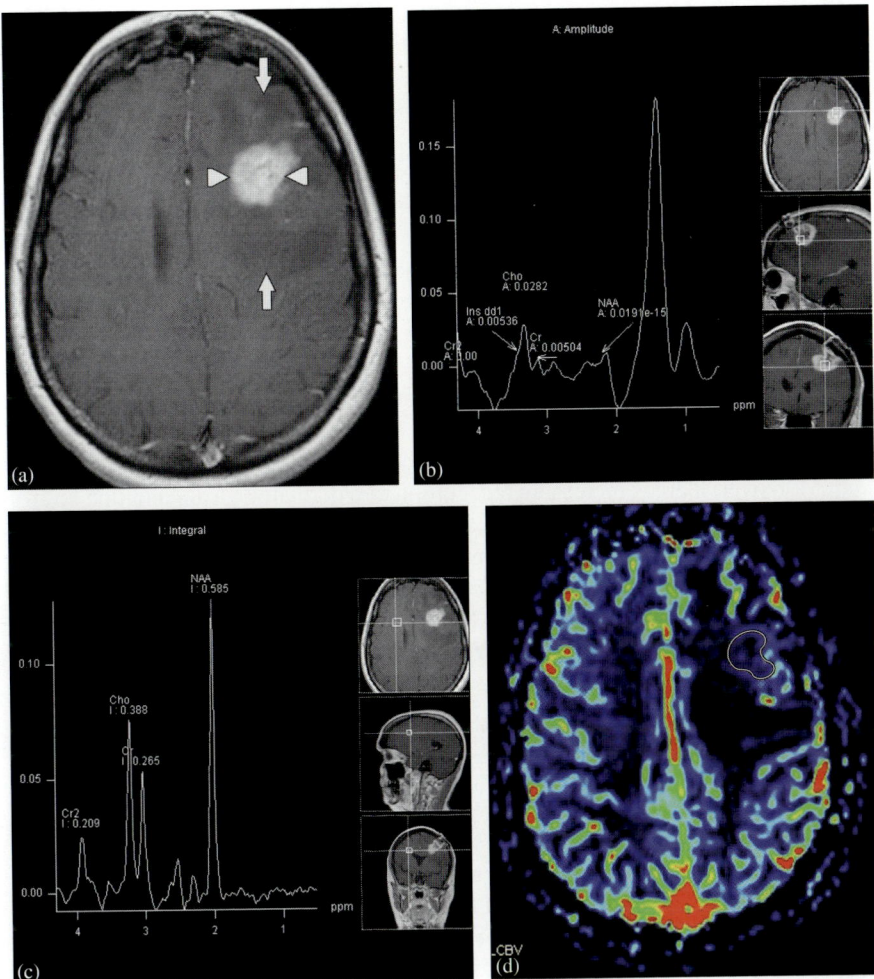

Figure 5. (a) **Radiation Necrosis**. Axial T1-weighted (MPRAGE) post-gadolinium image shows an enhancing lesion (arrowheads) in the left frontal lobe. Non-enhancing T1-hypointensity (arrows) represents edema. (b) MR Spectroscopy (single voxel, long TE = 144 ms) shows a classic profile for radiation necrosis that includes a markedly elevated lipid/lactate peak (broad peak from 0.9 to 1.4 ppm). Other peaks that are typically identifiable are lost in background noise (NAA, Cho, Cr). (c) MR Spectroscopy (single voxel, long TE = 144 ms) of contralateral normal white matter in the same patient shows a normal spectral pattern. (d) MR Perfusion (contrast-enhanced, echo-planar gradient echo technique) CBV parametric map identifies normal to low CBV corresponding to the enhancing lesion. The rCBV ratio compared to contralateral white matter is no greater than 1:1, compatible with radiation necrosis.

Magnetization transfer is a technique that suppresses background T1 hyperintensity in the brain parenchyma, improves lesion conspicuity and increase lesion counts [30]. The addition of an MT pulse may compete with non-MT higher contrast dose protocols [31]. There are drawbacks including a time-penalty and increased background noise.

Contrast agent properties germane to metastatic brain tumor imaging include intrinsic T1-relaxivity and user-defined elements such as dose and timing of post contrast imaging. Competition among contrast vendors is sharpening in the area of T1-relaxivity. A newer agent on the market (gadobenate dimeglumine) has the best T1-relaxivity, which relates to brightness on T1-weighted imaging, and has been shown in early work to improve lesion conspicuity [32]. Additional study is necessary to investigate the potential clinical impact of this property.

There remains debate over optimum contrast dose with a range of "single-dose" (0.1 mm/kg) to "triple-dose" (0.3 mm/kg) studies. Although some studies have shown improved lesion conspicuity with triple-dose, the financial impact is not small [33]. Moreover, there is increasing recognition of a dermatological condition known as nephrogenic systemic fibrosis that appears to occur in renal failure patients who have received "high-dose" gadolinium [34]. Finally, improvements in T1-relaxivity combined with other techniques such as MT may decrease or eliminate the "high-dose" advantage.

In general, delayed scanning after gadolinium administration is preferred to increase the conspicuity and lesion count in the case of metastasis [35]. The practical range that balances improved lesion detection against untenable time delays is ~5–15 minutes. One strategy that is employed is to administer contrast, run your T2 scan followed by your post-contrast T1 scan. Gadolinium does not affect T2 relaxation times and therefore this strategy provides the time delay without a true time penalty. Other factors that affect timing have been alluded to above including pulse sequence selection (i.e. 2D, 3D) and parameters (i.e. MT pulse), contrast dose and intrinsic contrast properties (i.e. T1-relaxivity) [36]. Field strength also plays a role particularly as 3 Tesla magnets become mainstream.

Perfusion Imaging

Perfusion imaging is a technique that displays physiological information of brain perfusion including cerebral blood volume (CBF, cc/100g of tissue), cerebral blood flow (CBV, cc/100g.min) and mean transit time (MTT, secs) [37]. These three parameters are related by the central volume principle and can be mathematically related (CBF = CBV/MTT). In brain tumor imaging, the parameter of interest is CBV because it relates to the status of neovascularity [38]. In the appropriate clinical setting, elevated CBV is consistent with tumor whereas diminished CBV can be seen in edematous brain parenchyma, radiation necrosis and infarct (Figs 4d, 5d) [39, 40].

Perfusion imaging can be performed by many modalities including MR, CT and nuclear medicine techniques. MR Perfusion is ideal for many reasons including whole brain coverage, improving spatial resolution, co-registration capabilities with other MR sequences and patient convenience. We prefer MR Perfusion for those reasons as well as the ability to quantify CBV (qCBV).

Quantifiable MR Perfusion was developed by Carroll et al. using a variety of techniques that include T1 mapping [41, 42]. This quantification can be applied to the two common MR Perfusion techniques: spin echo (SE) and gradient echo(GE). Both sequences have their strengths and weakness, which can be optimized depending upon the clinical scenario. Spin echo MRP accurately estimates qCBV but is better at the cortex due to fewer susceptibility effects from cortical vessels. Gradient echo MRP accurately estimates qCBV but is more sensitive to changes in the white matter and basal ganglion. Both techniques are quantifiable, which is important in the follow-up of treated lesions. If only qualitative analysis is available, common practice is to compare the relative CBV (rCBV) of the target lesion to normal appearing contralateral white matter. The higher the rCBV ratio, the more likely the lesion is neoplastic.

MR Perfusion can be used in a variety of settings including assessment of a solitary lesion, effects of systemic therapy and follow-up after surgery and radiation therapy to asses for radiation necrosis. When assessing a solitary lesion, CBV should be determined in the lesion itself and in the adjacent parenchyma: peritumoral edema from a metastasis will have a very low CBV (rCBV = 0.39 +/− 0.19) whereas infiltrating glioma will have elevated CBV (rCBV = 1.31 +/− 0.97) [43]. There is no statistical difference in CBV in infiltrating gliomas compared to parenchymal metastasis [43]. While undergoing chemotherapy, CBV can be tracked to assess the effects of treatment on neovascularity [44]. Once a lesion has undergone surgery and radiation therapy, recurrent enhancement is a dilemma: does this represent residual/recurrent tumor or radiation necrosis? Although not binary, radiation necrosis tends to have very low CBV (rCBV < 0.6) whereas tumor will have elevated CBV (rCBV >2.6) [40].

MR Spectroscopy

Spectroscopy is an MR technique used to investigate metabolic characteristics of a lesion. MRS is technically challenging pulse sequence and resource intensive. MRS can be acquired in 2D or 3D mode, as single voxel or multivoxel with short or long echo times all aimed at exploiting the different chemical shift properties of brain metabolites. These cases are typically monitored by a neuroradiologist and post-processing can be intensive. MRS cannot be interpreted in a vacuum and is best paired with MRP and conventional pulse sequences including FLAIR and post-contrast T1.

MRS can detect a range of spectra including normal brain, brain tumor, metastasis, radiation necrosis and vasogenic edema/gliosis (Figs 4b, 4c, 5b, 5c) [45]. Although some spectral patterns of enhancing neoplasm have been suggested to distinguish a metastatic lesion from a primary glial neoplasm (higher choline:creatine ratio), the sensitivity and specificity are not yet determined [43]. Spectral patterns of adjacent T2 signal abnormality are more likely to distinguish a metastasis from an infiltrating glioma because metastases are typically well-encapsulated or demarcated from adjacent brain parenchyma [43]. MRS is also useful, combined with MRP, in determining the presence of radiation necrosis versus residual/recurrent tumor [40].

Nuclear Medicine

The role of nuclear medicine techniques in the initial assessment of brain metastasis is limited, except for lymphoma versus toxoplasmosis in an immunocompromised patient. In patients with brain metastases, the primary niche for techniques that use radiotracers is the post-treatment setting to determine recurrent tumor from radiation necrosis. These techniques generally suffer from poor spatial resolution but benefit from intrinsic metabolic differences between tissues. The primary modalities are single photon emission computed tomography (SPECT) and positron emission tomography (PET).

SPECT Thallium-201

Thallium-201 (^{201}Tl) has biological properties similar to potassium and has been extensively used in cardiac imaging. ^{201}Tl does not cross the blood-brain-barrier and therefore does not typically accumulate in the brain parenchyma. Uptake in brain tumors is multifactorial and includes entering a cell via the sodium-potassium pump, leakiness due to intrinsic neovascularity properties and flow [46]. Although ^{201}Tl can be taken up by metastasis, sensitivity is low (approximately 70%) compared to MRI and not necessary for the diagnosis [47]. After treatment, ^{201}Tl can be used to distinguish recurrent tumor from radiation necrosis because necrosis does not exhibit uptake whereas tumor does [48]. That said, it is best to identify tumor recurrence early, which invariably means when the enhancement is very small: this requirement plus the relatively poor spatial resolution of ^{201}Tl SPECT limit its' usefulness. Combining ^{201}Tl SPECT with a perfusion technique such as 99m Tc-HMPAO or more recently, CT Perfusion or MR Perfusion, holds promise.

   In the immuncompromised population, specifically AIDS, the differential diagnosis for an enhancing intra-axial mass lesion includes lymphoma and abscess due to toxoplasmosis. Therapy for these two entities is disparate distinguishing between the two is important. In this population use of ^{201}Tl SPECT can help establish the diagnosis because lymphoma exhibits avid ^{201}Tl uptake whereas toxoplasmosis does not [49].

SPECT ^{99m}TcMIBI

Technitium 99m methoxyisobutylisonitrile (^{99m}Tc MIBI) was developed for cardiac perfusion imaging and was incidentally noted to have uptake in brain tumors [50]. Subsequent work showed sensitivity and specificity similar to that of ^{201}Tl in the detection of primary and metastatic brain tumors [47, 51]. Using early washout ratios, Yamamoto et al have shown sensitivity, specificity and accuracy of ^{99m}Tc MIBI of 93%, 83% and 90% [52]. Despite different mechanisms of uptake, early wash-out ratios for ^{201}Tl were identical; however, the average lesion-to-noise ratios were significantly higher for ^{99m}Tc MIBI. Normal uptake by the choroid plexus is a drawback of ^{99m}Tc MIBI although it produces sharper images, has lower background activity and has optimal photopeak energy compared to ^{201}Tl.

SPECT with Radiolabeled Amino Acids

Due to increased protein synthesis in tumor cells, radiolabeled amino acids such as iodomethyltyrosine (IMT) are taken up by tumor cells. This property has been used in combination with SPECT imaging to assess tumor grade and differentiate tumor from radiation necrosis with some success [53]. Clinical data remains limited and its' utility is not yet been fully established.

PET FDG

Radiolabeled fluorodeoxyglucose (FDG) is similar to glucose and is used as an indicator of glucose metabolism [54]. FDG is transported into the cell and is phosphorylated into FDG-6-phosphate, a monophasic derivative that cannot enter glycolysis and does not get transported out of the cell. Trapped in the cell, its accumulation is a marker for glucose metabolism. As radiotracers go, FDG is available and not exorbitantly expensive. It also has a workable half-life of just less than 2 hours (~100 minutes). The accessibility of FDG combined with the fact that brain tumors are hypermetabolic make FDG a realistic and practical radiotracer.

As with SPECT imaging, the utility of PET imaging for the diagnosis of brain metastasis is limited [55, 56]. Due to poor sensitivity and the typical small size of potential recurrent tumor, PET is of limited value in the setting of radiation necrosis versus recurrence.

Special Circumstances

Solitary Lesion

A solitary brain lesion has a broad differential including metastasis, primary brain tumor, abscess, stroke, hematoma and demyelination. In the setting of systemic tumor, a metastasis is the primary consideration. A critical step in this analysis is to be sure it's a solitary lesion. Was a 3D GE T1 used for post-contrast imaging? Does your tumor protocol address the issues of single dose versus higher dose gadolinium, implement magnetization transfer, acknowledge T1 relaxivity effects and consider delay from injection to T1 imaging? Are you certain these are not blood products or enhancement from a subacute stroke? The second step is to use everything in the imaging armamentarium to characterize the lesion. Is it hemorrhagic? Does it restrict diffusion? What are its T2 properties? Is melanin present? Does MRP confirm a hypervascular lesion with elevated CBV? Can MRS increase diagnostic confidence from the spectral characteristics of the lesion and adjacent brain? Finally, the location of white matter tracts can be assessed for pre-operative planning.

Steroids

A critical piece of the patient's history is whether they had been receiving steroids before or at the time of their imaging. The effect and mechanism of systemic steroid therapy on the enhancing characteristics of intra-axial metastases, peritumoral edema and whole brain perfusion have not been entirely elucidated but there are some trends that are important to consider. For example, it has been shown that T1-uptake (enhancement) in a small series of primary gliomas decreased 28% after 3 days of systemic dexamethasone therapy [57]. In the same study, a reduction in cerebral blood volume was identified in contralateral normal appearing white matter. In a separate study, blood flow to peritumoral edematous brain was shown to increase by 11.6% after similar therapy [58]. The mechanisms of these changes are not fully understood but relate in part to stabilization of the blood-tumor-barrier, decreased vascular permeability yielding less peritumoral edema and thus less local mass effect, in addition to the generalized vasoconstrictive action of steroids on the cerebral vasculature. These factors are important to consider when interpreting conventional MR imaging and advanced applications such as MR Perfusion

Post-Treatment Evaluation

In the setting of a metastatic disease that has undergone surgical resection, the post-operative imaging evaluation is focused on residual/recurrent tumor. In the subacute phase (up to 3 months post-operative), enhancing subacute infarction must be distinguished from recurrent tumor. Aside from comparing a post-operative DWI sequence to a subsequent enhanced scan, MRP and MRS can be helpful in determining dead tissue that is enhancing (stroke) from viable tissue that is enhancing (tumor, radiation necrosis). Long term post-operative follow-up utilizes a combination of conventional imaging characteristics, CBV estimates and spectral analyses to distinguish recurrent tumor from radiation necrosis. In some circumstances, ^{201}Tl SPECT or early wash-out ratios of ^{99m}Tc MIBI SPECT might have added value. These evaluations are among the most difficult and require consistent imaging parameters, in-house expertise and coordinated discussions with neuro-oncology and neurosurgery.

Brain Metastases without a Known Primary

Approximately 5–10% of patients with brain metastasis will not have a clear primary tumor [59]. Autopsy studies have found that bronchial carcinoma constitutes approximately 50% of these cases [60]. In this circumstance, specific characteristics of the lesions can be used to narrow the differential diagnosis but ultimately a full clinical work-up will be necessary to diagnose and treat the disease. The initial imaging work-up might include a CT scan of the chest, abdomen and pelvis but will be largely driven by the history, physical exam, blood work and clinical judgment.

References

1. Landis SH, Murray T, Bolden S et al. Cancer Statistics, 1998. CA Cancer J Clin 1999;49:8–31.
2. Posner J. Management of central nervous system metastases. Semin Oncol 1977;4:81–91
3. Vieth RG, Odom GL. Intracranial metastases and their neurosurgical treatment. J Neurosurg 1965;23:375–383
4. Egelhoff JC, Ross JS, Modic MT et al. MR imaging of metastatic GI adenocarcinoma in brain. AJNR 1992;13:1221–1224
5. Slimane, K, Andre F, Delaloge, S. Risk factors for brain relapse in patients with metastatic breast cancer. Ann Oncol 2004; 15:1640
6. Paulino AC, Nguyen TX, Barker JL. Brain metastasis in children with sarcoma, neuroblastoma and Wilms' tumor. Int. J Radiation Oncology Bio Phys. 2003;57(1):177–183
7. Clouston PD, DeAngelis LM, Posner JB. The spectrum of neurological disease in patients with systemic cancer. Ann Neurol 1992;31(3):268–273.
8. Walter BA, Valera VA, Takahashi S et al. the olfactory route for cerebrospinal fluid drainage into the peripheral lymphatic system. Neuropathol Appl Neurobiol. 2006 Aug;32(4):388–396.
9. Patchell RA. Brain metastases. Neurol Clin 1991;9:817–824.
10. Bruner JM, Tien RD. Secondary tumors. In: Russell DS, Rubenstein LJ (editors). Pathology of tumors of the nervous system, 6th edition. Baltimore, Williams and Wilkins, 1997;419–450.
11. Henson RA, Urich H. Metastases to the Brian. In: Henson RA, Urich H. Cancer of the nervous system. The neurological manifestations of systemic malignant disease. Oxford: Blackwell Scientific, 1982;7–58.
12. Lantos PL, Louis DN, Rosenblum MK et al. Tumours of the nervous system. In: Graham DI, Lantos PL, editors. Greenfield's Neuropathology, 7th ed. London: Arnold, 2002:11;767–1052.

13. Pathak AP, Schmainda KM, Ward BD et al. MR-derived cerebral blood volume maps: issues regarding histological validation and assessment of tumor angiogenesis. Magn Reson Med 2001;46(4):735–747.

14. Law M, Yang S, Babb JS et al. Comparison of cerebral blood volume and vascular permeability from dynamic susceptibility contrast-enhanced perfusion MR imaging with glioma grade. Am J Neuroradiol 2004;25:746–755

15. Nutt SH, Patchell RA. Intracranial hemorrhage associated with primary and secondary tumors. Neurosurg Clin 1992;3:591–599.

16. Davis PC, Hudgins PA, Peterman SB et al. Diagnosis of cerebral metastasis: double-dose delayed CT vs. contrast-enhanced MR imaging. Am J Neuroradiol 1991;12:293–300.

17. Schellinger PD, Meinck HM, Thron A. Diagnostic accuracy of MRI compared to CC in patients with brain metastases. Journal of Neuro-Oncolgy 1999;44:275–281.

18. Komiyama M, Yagura H, Baba M et al. MR imaging: possibility of tissue characterization of brain tumors using T1 and T2 values. Am J Neuroradiol 1987;8:65–70.

19. Komara J, Nayini N, Bialick H et al. Brain iron delocalization and lipid peroxidation following cardiac arrest. Ann Emerg Med 1986;15:384–389.

20. Partovi S, Fram EK, Karis JP. Fast Spin Echo MR Imaging. Neuroimaging Clin N Am 1999;9(3):553–576.

21. Stevenson VL, Gawne-Cain ML, Barker GJ et al. Imaging of the spinal cord and brain in multiple sclerosis. a comparative study between fast flair and fast pin echo. J Neurol 1997;244:119–124.

22. Atlas SW, Thulborn KR. Intracranial hemorrhage. In: Atlas SW, editor. Magnetic Resonance Imaging of the Brain and Spine, 3rd edition. Philadelphia, Lippincott, Williams and Wilkins, 2002:773–832.

23. Schaefer PW, Copen WA, Lev M et al. Diffusion-weighted imaging in acute stroke. Neuroimaging Clin N Am 2005;15(3):503–530.

24. Rowley HA, Grant PE, Roberts TPL. Diffusion MR imaging: Theory and applications. Neuroimaging Clin N Am 1999;9(2):343–362.

25. Gupta RK, Sinha U, Cloughesy TF et al. Inverse correlation between choline magnetic resonance spectroscopy signal intensity and the apparent diffusion coefficient in human glioma. Magn Reson Med 1999;41(1):2–7

26. Camacho DL, Smith JK, Castillo M. Differentiation of toxoplasmosis and lymphoma in AIDS patients by using apparent diffusion coefficients. Am J Neuroradiol 2003;24(4):633–637

27. Hayashida Y, Hirai T, Morishita et al. Diffusion-weighted imaging of metastatic brain tumors: Comparison with histologic type and tumor cellularity. Am J Neuroradiol 2006; 27:1419–25.

28. Price SJ, Jena R, Burnet NG et al. Improved delineation of glioma margins and regions of infiltration with the use of diffusion tensor imaging: An image-guided biopsy study. Am J Neuroradiol 2006;27:1969–1974.

29. Brant-Zawadzki M, Gillan GD, Nitz WR. MP RAGE: A three-dimensional, T1-weighted, gradient-echo sequence-Initial experience in the brain. Radiol 1992;182:769–775.
30. Finelli DA, Hurst GC, Gullapalli RP et al. T1-weighted three-dimensional magnetization transfer MR of the brain: improved lesion contrast enhancement. Am J Neuroradiol 1998;19:59–64.
31. Knauth M, Forsting M, Hartman M et al. MR enhancement of brain lesions: increased contrast dose compared with magnetization transfer. Am J Neuroradiol 1996;17:1853–1859
32. Maravilla KR, Maldjian JA, Schmalfuss IM et al. Contrast enhancement of central nervous system lesions: Multicenter intraindividual crossover comparative study of two MR contrast agents. Radiol 2006; 240(2):398–400.
33. Yuh WTC, Engelken JD, Muhonen MC et al. Experience with high-dose gadolinium MR imaging in the evaluation of brain metastases. Am J Neuroradiol 1992;13:335–345.
34. Kuo PH, Kanal E, Abu-Alfa AK et al. Gadolinium-based MR contrast agents and nephrogenic systemic fibrosis. Radiol 2007 (Jan);[Epub ahead of print].
35. Grzesiakowska U, Tachikowska M. An assessment of the effectiveness of magnetic resonance imaging in delayed sequences after administration of Gd-DTPA contrast in the detection of metastatic lesions. Med Sci Monit 2002;8(1):21–4.
36. Yuh WTC, Tali ET, Nguyen HD et al. the effect of contrast dose, imaging time, and lesion size in the MR detection of intracerebral metastasis. Am J Neuroradiol 1995;16:373–380.
37. Wintermark M, Sesay M, Barbier E et al. Comparative overview of brain perfusion imaging techniques. J Neuroradiol 2005;32(5):294–314.
38. Aronen HJ, Pardo FS, Kennedy DN, et al. High microvascular blood volume is associated with high glucose uptake and tumor angiogenesis in human gliomas. Clin Cancer Res 2000;6(6): 2189–2200.
39. Uematsu H, Maeda M, Itoh H. Peritumoral brain edema in intracranial meningiomas evaluated by dynamic perfusion-weighted MR imaging: a preliminary study. Eur Radiol 2003;13(4):758–762.
40. Sugahara T, Korogi Y, Tomiguchi S et al. Post-therapeutic intra-axial brain tumor: the value of perfusion sensitive contrast-enhanced MR imaging for differentiating tumor recurrence from nonneoplastic contrast-enhancing tumor. Am J Neuroradiol 2000;21(5):901–909.
41. Sakaie KE, Shin W, Curtin KR et al. Method for improving the accuracy of quantitative cerebral perfusion imaging. J Magn Reson Imaging 2005;21(5):512–519.
42. Shin W, Cashen TA, Horowitz SW et al. Quantitative CBV measurement form static T1 changes in tissue and correction for intravascular water exchange. Magn Reson Med 2006;56(1):138–145.

43. Law M, Cha S, Knopp EA, Johnson G, Arnett J, Litt AW. High-grade gliomas and solitary metastases: differentiation by using perfusion and proton spectroscopic MR imaging. Radiol 2002; 222(3):715–721.

44. Cha S, Knopp EA, Johnson G et al. Dynamic contrast-enhanced T2-weighted MR imaging of recurrent malignant gliomas treated with thalidomide and carboplatin. Am J Neuroradiol 2000;21(5):881–890.

45. Al-Okaili RN, Krejza J, Wang S et al. Advanced MR imaging techniques in the diagnosis of intra-axial brain tumors in adults. Radiographics 2006;26(S1):73–89.

46. Schillaci Orazio, Filippi L, Manni C et al. Single-Photon emission computed tomography/computed tomography in brain tumors. Semin Nucl Med 2007;37:34–47.

47. Kashitani N, Makihara S, Maeda T et al. Thallium-201-chloride and technetium-99m-MIBI SPECT of primary and metastatic lung carcinoma. Oncol Rep 1999;6(1):127–133.

48. Datta NR, Pasricha R, Gambhir S et al. Comparative evaluation of Tl-201 SPECT and CT in the follow-up of irradiated brain tumors. Int J Clin Oncol 2004;9:51–58.

49. Lorberboym M, Estok L, Machac J et al. Rapid differential diagnosis of cerebral toxoplasmosis and primary central nervous system lymphoma by thallium-201 SPECT. J Nucl Med 1996;37(7):1150–1154.

50. O'Tuama LA, Packard AB, Treves ST: SPECT imaging of pediatric brain tumor with hexakis (methoxyisobutylisonitrile) technetium (I). J Nucl Med 1990;31:2040–2041.

51. O'Tuama LA, Treves ST, Larar JN et al. Thallium-201 versus technetium-99m-MIBI SPECT in evaluation of childhood brain tumors. A within subject comparison. J Nucl Med 1993;34:1045–1051.

52. Yamamoto Y, Nishiyama Y, Toyama Y et al. 99mTc-MIBI and 201Th SPET in the detection of recurrent brain tumours after radiation therapy. Nucl Med Commun 2002;23:1183–1190.

53. Benard F, Romsa J, Hustinx R. Imaging gliomas with positron emission tomography and single-photon emission computed tomography. Semin Nucl Med 2003;33(2):148–162.

54. Hustinx R, Alavi A. SPECT and PET imaging of brain tumors. Neuroimaging Clin N Am 1999;9(4):751–766.

55. Posther KE, McCall LM, Harpole DH et al. Yield of Brain 18F-FDG PET in evaluating patients with potentially operable non-small cell lung cancer. J Nucl Med 2006;47(10):1607–1611

56. Rohren EM, Provenzale JM, Barboriak DP et al. Screening for cerebral metastases with FDG PET in patients undergoing whole-body staging of non-central nervous system malignancy. Radiology 2003;226: 181–187.

57. Wilkinson ID, Jellineck DA, Levy D et al. Dexamethasone and enhancing solitary cerebral mass lesions: alterations in perfusion and blood-tumor barrier kinetics shown by magnetic resonance imaging. Neurosurgery 2006;58:640–646.
58. Bastin ME, Carpenter TK, Armitage PA. Effects of dexamethasone on cerebral perfusion and water diffusion in patients with high-grade glioma. Am J Neuro-radiol 2006;27:402–408.
59. Delattre JY, Krol G, Thaler HT et al. Distribution of brain metastases. Arch Neurol 1988;45:741–744.
60. Deangelis LM. Management of brain metastases. Cancer Invest 1994;12: 156–165.

4. SYMPTOM MANAGEMENT AND SUPPORTIVE CARE OF THE PATIENT WITH BRAIN METASTASES

Herbert B. Newton, M.D., FAAN

Abstract

The focus of care for patients with brain metastases will always be on thera-peutic options such as surgery, radiotherapy, and chemotherapy. However, proper symptom management and supportive care of non-therapeutic issues will be equally as important, including treatment of seizures, use of anticonvulsants, corticosteroids, and gastric acid inhibitors, assessment of swallowing dysfunction, treatment of thromboembolic events, appropriate use and safe application of anticoagulation, and evaluation of psychiatric issues. Appropriate management of these supportive aspects of patient care will improve overall quality of life and allow the patient and family to more easily concentrate on treatment.

Introduction

The modern treatment of patients with metastatic brain tumors (MBT) usually involves a team approach from a dedicated group of physicians, nurses, and support staff that specialize in various aspects of neuro-oncology, along with a Tumor Board specific for neuro-oncology patients [1]. Although the focus of the treatment team will be on therapeutic strategies to control tumor growth (e.g., surgical resection, radiotherapy, chemotherapy), many other facets of care are necessary and will involve patient support and symptom management, in an effort to maintain quality of life. The challenge for the treatment team begins at the moment of diagnosis, when the bad news must be communicated to the patient and family. Recent research suggests there are several important factors that should be considered when imparting a new cancer diagnosis [2]. It is critical that the physician use simple, non-technical language in a non-patronizing manner, with a warm and caring tone. Every effort should be made to empathize with the emotions the patient is experiencing. The physician should sit close to the patient and maintain good eye contact. It is also permissible to initiate physical contact, in an effort to provide comfort. A quiet, private, and comfortable room should be used for the meeting, where interruptions and distractions can be minimized. Many patients also find it helpful when the physician gives some kind of warning that bad news is forthcoming and does not rush through the ensuing discussion. In addition, the physician must accurately gauge how explicit to be in terms of information regarding prognosis in the context of neuro-oncologic disease. Some patients and families are medically sophisticated and well read, and realize the prognosis for longterm survival is typically poor [3]. In contrast, other patients and families are ambivalent or actively disinterested in learning about the poor prognosis associated with their disease [4]. Each of these disparate situations will require a different approach by the physician, as the groundwork for active treatment is negotiated.

The role of support is crucial for MBT patients and their families, and continues until the patient is cured or, more often, succumbs to their disease [5]. The most important initial form of support is information and education about the diagnosis. At the moment the patient and family hear the words "brain tumor", they enter into a crisis mode and often feel a loss of control, fear of the unknown, and sense of helplessness. To regain some aspect of control of their lives, they need to learn as much as possible about the disease and form a partnership with their physician, taking an aggressive and active role in the plan for treatment and recovery. Informational brochures and other written materials are helpful, as are the websites of organizations that provide services and resources for patients and families, such as the North American Brain Tumor Coalition [5]. The Coalition is a network of charitable organizations dedicated to the cure of brain tumors, and includes the American Brain Tumor Association, the Brain Tumor Foundation for Children, the Brain Tumor Foundation of Canada, The Brain Tumor Society, The Children's Brain Tumor Foundation, the National Brain Tumor Foundation, the Pediatric Brain Tumor Foundation of the United States, and the Preuss Foundation. During the course of a devastating illness such as metastatic brain cancer, the patient's family will usually be the greatest source of support and comfort, as well as active caregivers in the home setting [5, 6]. In this context, family members often take on the role of information seekers and patient advocates. It is important to note that family caregivers are also at risk for depression and other signs of stress, and require a strong support network to function effectively in this role [7]. Other sources of support for the patient and caregivers include the nurses of the treatment team, oncological social workers, Chaplains affiliated with the hospital or from the private sector, and hospital-based support groups (brain tumor specific or general).

The remaining sections of this chapter will review the various aspects of supportive care that may be necessary in the management of MBT patients.

Seizures and Anticonvulsant Therapy

Seizure activity is a frequent complication in brain tumor patients and often compromises quality of life by the restriction of driving privileges, through seizure-related injuries, loss of time at work, and anxiety related to subsequent ictal events [8]. In addition, quality of life can be further affected by the side effects, drug interactions, and expenses incurred by the use of antiepileptic drugs (AED). Seizures occur at presentation in 20% to 40% of patients with MBT [8, 9]. It is important to note that more than 25% of adults between 25 and 64 years of age with newly diagnosed seizures will have an underlying brain tumor [8]. At the time of neurological disease progression, seizure activity often becomes more frequent and severe, affecting another 10% to 20% of patients. Younger patients (e.g., children and young adults), tend to have a higher incidence of seizure activity when tumor involvement is supratentorial in location. In general, supratentorial tumors are most likely to cause seizures, especially when located within or near the cortex. Multifocal or bihemispheric tumors are also known to cause frequent ictal events. Seizures are much less common with tumors that are deep-seated or confined to the white matter.

Patients with less infiltrative and irritative brain involvement typically manifest seizures that are equally divided between partial motor, partial complex, and secondarily generalized varieties [8, 9]. For patients with MBT, focal motor seizures are the predominant variety, with less common secondarily generalized and complex partial seizures. The neurological examination can be relatively normal and nonfocal in some MBT patients with seizures. However, the majority of these patients will have seizure activity associated with focal neurological deficits on examination [8, 9].

The pathophysiological mechanisms underlying tumor-associated seizures (TAS) remain unclear [8–11]. Recent evidence using direct brain recordings of electrical activity suggest that TAS originate from intact, non-infiltrated, neural tissue adjacent to tumors, and not from within the tumor mass itself [10]. Histologically, epileptogenic regions of brain demonstrate gliosis and mild reactive astrocytosis, without evidence for tumor cells. It is now theorized that these peritumoral epileptogenic foci develop an imbalance between excitatory and inhibitory inputs, due to multifactorial alterations in the local milieu from the tumor. The intra- and extracellular pH is slightly alkaline in peritumoral tissues, which enhances excitatory neuronal pathways and induces a 30% reduction of activity in GABAergic inhibitory pathways [10]. In biopsy samples from peritumoral epileptic foci, the number of GABA- and somatostatin-containing neurons are decreased [12]. Similar biopsy studies have noted an elevated concentration of glutamine, the direct precursor of glutamate, in peritumoral epileptogenic foci of gliomas [13]. Glutamine is taken up and secreted by normal glia and glioma cells, thus providing a large reservoir of precursor for peritumoral neurons to convert to glutamate. In addition, recent evidence suggests that glioma cells directly secrete glutamate, causing significantly increased, excitotoxic concentrations in peritumoral tissues [14, 15]. In vitro experiments have demonstrated extensive NMDA and AMPA receptor stimulation and delayed Ca^{2+}-dependent cell death in exposed neurons. These reports suggest that exposure of peritumoral neurons to chronically elevated concentrations of glutamate could contribute to neuronal injury, abnormalities of neuronal circuitry, and the development of epileptiform activity. It remains unclear if tumor cells from MBT are capable of glutamate secretion. Other peritumoral alterations that may contribute to epileptogenic potential include increased extracellular Fe^{3+}, dysfunction of astrocytic syncytial gap junctions due to the infiltration of tumor cells, and the presence of pro-inflammatory cytokines (e.g., TNF-α), which can increase membrane excitability.

The diagnosis of a seizure in a MBT patient is usually a clinical diagnosis, based on the history and description of the symptom complex from the patient and family members [8, 9]. Testing with routine electroencephalography (EEG) is not helpful in most patients, since only 25% to 33% will demonstrate any focal interictal epileptiform activity. Prolonged EEG monitoring (with or without a video component) may be more helpful in diagnosing seizures in confusing or subtle cases. In one half of the active seizure group, ictal events will occur more than once per month, while another 25% will have events more than once per week, despite the use of AED. The presence of seizure activity does not impact on the overall survival of brain tumor patients [8]. However, patients that present with a seizure may have a more favorable prognosis. The most likely explanation for this phenomenon is that seizures will often lead to a more prompt work-up and earlier diagnosis, when the tumor burden is smaller and more amenable to therapy. Patients with chronic seizures that develop a new pattern, with frequent "breakthrough" activity, may relate to a change in the tumor such as bleeding or dedifferentiation into a more rapidly growing and more malignant lesion. It is also possible to have a "flare-up" of seizure activity, in otherwise well-controlled patients, at the onset of certain therapies that may cause irritation to surrounding brain, such as at the initiation of external beam radiotherapy and with certain forms of chemotherapy (e.g., gliadel wafers, intra-arterial cisplatin).

There is general consensus that any MBT patient with a well documented, unequivocal seizure (generalized or focal) should be placed on an AED (see Table 1) [8, 9, 10]. For adult patients with generalized seizures, phenytoin, carbamazepine, and valproate have relatively equivalent efficacy for reducing seizure activity [16, 17]. Similarly, all three drugs are effective for partial motor, partial sensory, and partial complex seizures. However, a comparative trial of carbamazepine and valproate has demonstrated better control of complex partial seizure activity with carbamazepine [18]. Monotherapy with phenytoin, carbamazepine, or valproate would be a reasonable choice for initial management in most patients [9, 16, 17]. In some patients, a second drug must be added if high therapeutic concentrations of several of the first line drugs are unable to control seizure activity. Phenytoin or carbamazepine in combination with valproate is a common strategy. Alternatively, one of the new generation anticonvulsants (e.g., levetiracetam, gabapentin,

Table 1. Antiepileptic Drugs Commonly Used for Treatment of Seizures in Brain Tumor Patients

Drug	Dose (mg/d)	Metabolism	Enzyme Inducing	Mechanism	Bound Fraction (%)
TRADITIONAL AED'S					
phenytoin	300–400	hepatic+++	+++	sodium channel	90–95
carbamazepine	800–1,600	hepatic+++	+++	sodium channel	75
valproic acid	1,000–3,000	hepatic+++	no; Inhibitory	sodium channel; enhanced GABA	80–90
phenobarbital	90–180	hepatic+++	+++	EAA antagonist; enhanced GABA	45
NEWER AED'S					
felbamate	2,400–3,600	hepatic++	+	EAA antagonist; enhanced GABA	25
lamotrigine	100–500	hepatic+++	none	sodium channel	55
gabapentin	1,800–3,600	renal+++	none	enhanced GABA	< 5
topiramate	200–400	hepatic+	none	sodium channel; EAA antagonist; enhanced GABA	9–17
tiagabine	32–56	hepatic+++	none	enhanced GABA	95
oxcarbazine	600–1,800	hepatic+++	+	sodium channel	40
levetiracetam	1,000–3,000	renal++	None	binding to synaptic vesicle protein SV2A; enhanced GABA; calcium channels	< 10
zonisamide	100–400	hepatic++	none	sodium& calcium channels; enhanced GABA	40

Adapted from references[8, 9, 10, 16, 21]
Abbreviations: mg/d – mg/day; AED – antiepileptic drug; + – mild; ++ – moderate; +++ – severe; EAA – excitatory amino acids; GABA - gamma amino butyric acid

topiramate, zonisamide) could be added to one of the first line agents [19–21]. Levetiracetam may be an excellent choice, since initial experience suggests it is effective and well tolerated in brain tumor patients, and has minimal potential to interact with other drugs such as corticosteroids or chemotherapy agents [21]. Ongoing studies will determine if levetiracetam and other new generation agents might be appropriate for first line monotherapy applications or as secondary, stand-alone agents. Serum drug concentrations should be monitored and optimized in all patients whenever appropriate (e.g., phenytoin, carbamazepine, valproate).

In the brain tumor population, seizures remain difficult to control despite the use of AED. Patients who present with seizures tend to be more refractory to therapy than those that develop seizures later in the course of their disease [8, 9]. In general, recurrent seizure activity is common, despite aggressive anticonvulsant therapy. Patient compliance can contribute to this problem and is frequently sub-optimal. In many patients with a recent seizure, anticonvulsant levels are subtherapeutic. Further complicating the situation is that brain tumor patients are more susceptible to AED toxicity and side effects, including cognitive impairment, hepatotoxicity, myelosuppression, skin rashes (including Stevens-Johnson syndrome), and interactions with concomitant medications [8]. Several of the AED (e.g., phenytoin, carbamazepine, phenobarbital) enhance hepatic microsomal P-450-mediated metabolism of concomitant medications. This is especially problematic for patients receiving chemotherapy (e.g., nitrosoureas, irinotecan, paclitaxel, methotrexate), leading to lower tissue concentrations and reduced efficacy [8, 22]. Some of the newer AED (e.g., levetiracetam, gabapentin) do not enhance the hepatic P-450 system and may be better choices in selected patients [21].

Anticonvulsant drugs are frequently administered to neuro-oncology patients at the time of diagnosis or after craniotomy, as prophylaxis for potential seizure activity [8]. This practice was given early support in the literature, despite the fact that the data in these reports was modest at best [23, 24]. All subsequent reports on the use of AED prophylaxis do not support this practice, including a randomized, blinded, placebo-controlled trial of valproate in patients with newly diagnosed MBT and PBT [25–29]. In this study, the odds ratio for a seizure in the valproate arm relative to the placebo arm was 1.7 (p = 0.3) [29]. Most authors would now recommend withholding implementation of AED in newly diagnosed brain tumor patients until a seizure has been documented. This approach is supported by a recent meta-analysis by Glantz and associates for the American Academy of Neurology [30]. In addition, for patients that have not had a seizure and have received AED for craniotomy, tapering and discontinuing the AED after the first postoperative week is recommended [30].

Corticosteroids

The use of corticosteroids is often necessary in MBT patients to control symptoms caused by increased intracranial pressure (e.g., headache, nausea and emesis, confusion, weakness) [9, 31]. Peritumoral edema is the principal cause of elevated intracranial pressure and is mediated through numerous mechanisms, including the leaky neovasculature associated with tumor angiogenesis, as well as increased permeability induced by factors secreted by the tumor and surrounding tissues, such as oxygen free radicals, arachidonic acid, glutumate, histamine, bradykinin, atrial natriuretic peptide, and vascular endothelial growth factor (VEGF) [32–34]. Dexamethasone is the high-potency steroid used most often to treat the edema associated with brain tumors [9, 31]. It has several advantages over other synthetic glucocorticoids, including a longer half-life, reduced mineralocorticoid effect, lower incidence of cognitive and behavioral complications, and diminished inhibition of leukocyte migration [35]. The mechanisms by which dexamethasone and other glucocorticoids reduce peritumoral edema remain unclear. It is known that MBT have high concentrations of glucocorticoid receptors. The effects of these drugs on tumor-induced edema are most likely mediated through binding to these receptors, with subsequent transfer to the nucleus and the expression of novel genes [34]. In a recent MRI study, dexamethasone was able to induce a dramatic reduction in blood-tumor barrier permeability and regional cerebral blood volume, without significant alteration of cerebral blood flow or the degree of edema [36]. The inhibition of production and/or release of vasoactive factors secreted by tumor cells and endothelial cells, such as VEGF and prostacyclin, appears to be involved in this process [33, 34]. In addition, glucocorticoids appear to inhibit the reactivity of endothelial cells to several substances that induce capillary permeability.

The exact dose of steroids necessary for each patient will vary depending on the neuro-oncological process, size and location of the tumor, if present, and amount of peritumoral edema. In general, most patients with MBT will require between 4 and 12 mg of dexamethasone per day to remain clinically stable. The lowest dose of steroid that can control the patient's pressure-related symptoms should be used [9, 31]. This approach will minimize some of the toxicity and complications that can arise from long-term corticosteroid usage, which includes hyperglycemia, peripheral edema, proximal myopathy, gastritis, infection, osteopenia, weight gain, bowel perforation, and psychiatric or behavioral changes (e.g., euphoria, hypomania, depression, psychosis, sleep disturbance)[9, 37–42]. Patients with dexamethasone-induced proximal myopathy will often improve when the dosage is reduced [41, 42]. In addition, the proximal leg muscles can usually be strengthened if the patient is placed on a lower extremity exercise regimen. Some authors have also reported an improvement in the myopathy when dexamethasone is replaced by an equivalent dosage of prednisone or hydrocortisone [41, 42]. The neuropsychiatric complications of steroids can often be improved by dosage reduction or discontinuation of the drug [40]. For those patients in whom continued steroid usage is necessary, symptomatic pharmacological intervention is appropriate. For example, patients experiencing steroid-induced delirium or psychosis will often improve with low-dose haloperidol (0.5 to 1.0 mg PO, IM, or IV), titrated to control symptoms. Steroid-induced sleep disturbances often respond to dosage reduction or by eliminating any doses after dinner. In refractory cases, the use of a hypnotic medication at bedtime (e.g., triazolam, 0.25 mg) will often be of benefit. Corticosteroid-induced osteoporosis is a common problem, affecting 30% to 50% of patients receiving treatment for a year or more [37, 43, 44]. Patients on long-term dexamethosone require a preventive program to minimize osteoporosis, including calcium and vitamin D supplements, and weight-bearing exercises. These measures should be started early, since bone loss is greatest in the first two to four months of chronic steroid treatment. For patients on long-term steroid therapy (i.e., $\geq$ 3 months), or in those with established osteoporosis or evidence of an osteoporotic fracture, bisphosphonate therapy (e.g., risedronate, 2.5–5.0 mg/day; alendronate, 5–10 mg/day) should be added to the regimen of calcium and vitamin D supplements [44].

Metastatic brain tumor patients can be immunosuppressed for a variety of reasons, including long-term steroid use, immunomodulatory factors secreted by the tumor, and the effects of chemotherapy [35, 37]. Chronic steroid usage can lead to lymphopenia, mainly through a reduction in the concentration of CD4+ T cells, and an associated increased risk of systemic infection. Recent studies suggest that brain tumor patients on chronic steroids are at substantial risk for pneumocystis carinii pneumonia (PCP), a serious infection with a 50% to 55% case fatality rate. In a recent pair of reports reviewing the Johns Hopkins experience over the past 20 years, Grossman and colleagues noted that the rate of PCP in brain tumor patients was less than 1.0% [45, 46]. However, of all HIV negative patients with PCP over the past five years, the percentage with brain tumors had increased from 22% to 40%. The authors did not recommend PCP prophylaxis for every brain tumor patient on long-term steroids or chemotherapy. Rather, they suggested careful monitoring of all patients for the onset of lymphopenia, including an assessment in high-risk cases of the concentration of CD4+ T cells. For those high-risk patients with lymphopenia and CD4 counts below 200 cells/mL, a prophylactic anti-PCP regimen should be instituted [46]. The most commonly used prophylactic antibiotic is trimethoprim-sulphamethoxazole (TMP-SMX, 160+800 mg), at a dose of one double strength tablet per day. For patients with a sulpha allergy or deleterious interactions between TMP-SMX and other drugs (e.g., methotrexate), alternative prophylactic medications include pentamidine (300 mg/month by nebulizer) and dapsone (100 mg/day by mouth).

Gastric Acid Inhibitors

Brain tumor patients on long-term dexamethasone are at increased risk for gastrointestinal complications (i.e., gastritis, ulceration, bowel perforation), although there remains some debate in the literature regarding ulcer formation [31, 37, 39]. A comprehensive review of the topic would suggest that ulcer prophylaxis is appropriate, since the incidence of ulcer formation is increased in patients with advanced malignant disease [47]. Patients at risk should be treated prophylactically with a gastric acid inhibitor such as ranitidine hydrochloride (150 mg po bid), famotidine (20 mg po bid), or omeprazole (20–40 mg po qd) [48, 49]. These medications can be discontinued after the patient has been completely tapered off dexamethasone.

Thromboembolic Complications & Anticoagulation

The risk of thromboembolism (i.e., deep venous thrombosis [DVT], pulmonary embolism [PE]) is high in cancer patients, with an antemortem incidence of symptomatic events approaching 15% [50–53]. However, at autopsy the incidence rates are much higher, between 45% and 50% in some series. For patients with brain tumors, the risk for DVT and PE appears to be even higher than the general cancer population [51, 53]. In the perioperative period, the overall incidence of thrombosis after brain tumor resection was 45%, as detected by ^{125}I-labeled fibrinogen scans [52]. The incidence varied depending on the tumor type, and was 20% for MBT patients. Thromboembolic risk continues to remain high in brain tumor patients after the perioperative period (i.e., beyond 6 weeks). For example, a meta-analysis of glioma patients noted a DVT incidence rate that ranged from 0.013 to 0.023 per patient-month of follow-up, corresponding to overall rates of 7% to 24% [54]. The only prospective study included in the analysis followed 75 patients until death and had a DVT incidence rate of 24% (0.015 DVT/patient-month) [55]. In addition to biological factors related to individual tumor histology, several clinical factors are also associated with increased risk of DVT and PE, including arm paresis, leg paresis, history of prior DVT or PE before tumor diagnosis, and longer operative time [53, 54, 56]. Other less important factors that may also be relevant are older age, larger tumor size, and the use of chemotherapy.

If a patient with a MBT develops a thromboembolic event, should they be treated with conventional anticoagulation approaches, or is that too dangerous and should they, instead, receive an inferior vena cava filter (VCF) without anticoagulation? The important question at the core of this dilemma is the risk of intra-tumoral hemorrhage while receiving anticoagulant therapy. This is a common problem for the neuro-oncology treatment team and continues to be studied in the literature. In general, the risk for symptomatic hemorrhage into a brain tumor is quite low during conservative anticoagulation with heparin and coumadin [53, 55–60]. Most authors report a hemorrhage rate of 5% to 7% for MBT. In order to minimize the potential for intra-tumoral hemorrhage, the parameters for heparin and coumadin therapy need to be very conservative, with PTT and PT values in the 1.5 to 2.0 times control range [56]. Once the patient has shifted completely over to coumadin, the INR should be maintained between 1.5 and 2.5 [53, 58].

A more recent approach to treating a thromboembolic event would be to use a low-molecular-weight heparin (LMWH) [50, 61]. The LMWH's (e.g., enoxaparin, dalteparin) are composed of fragments of unfractionated heparin produced by controlled enzymatic or chemical depolymerization, yielding chains with an average molecular weight of 5000 daltons. In comparison to unfractionated heparin, LMWH's have a more predictable anticoagulant response due to better bioavailability, a longer half-life, and more dose-dependent clearance [61]. In addition, the LMWH's can be administered subcutaneously in the outpatient setting and do not require monitoring of coagulation status. When used in clinical trials of patients with deep venous thrombosis, LMWH's (e.g., enoxaparin, 100 U/kg twice daily) have proved as effective or more effective than unfractionated heparin, with a lower hemorrhage rate [61]. Meta-analyses of the clinical trial data conclude, in general, that LMWH's are more effective and safer than unfractionated heparin. However, the above mentioned studies have not included brain tumor patients. Clinical trials to more specifically evaluate the safety and efficacy of LMWH in brain tumor patients have not been completed.

The utility of VCF in brain tumor patients remains controversial [62]. Several studies have demonstrated a significant complication rate for VCF in PBT and MBT patients (range 40% to 62%) and suggest that biological factors related to the tumor may be involved [59, 60]. Complications after VCF placement include filter thrombosis, recurrent DVT, recurrent PE, and thrombosis of the inferior vena cava. Patients receiving anticoagulation had a lower recurrence rate of PE and DVT. Although most authors now suggest that acute and long-term anticoagulation is superior to VCF placement for brain tumor patients with DVT and/or PE, selected patients should still be considered for this approach. Patients with large regions of intra-tumoral hemorrhage, impaired neurological function and excessive risk for falling episodes, and gastrointestinal bleeding should be evaluated for VCF placement instead of anticoagulation.

Dysphagia & Swallowing Disorders

Dysphagia and disorders of swallowing are common in patients with neurological disease, and can be associated with stroke, multiple sclerosis, motor neuron disease, neurodegenerative disorders, and structural lesions such as a PBT or MBT [63–69]. Swallowing dysfunction can lead to serious morbidity from malnutrition, dehydration, and aspiration pneumonia. There remains a paucity of literature regarding the incidence and presentation of dysphagia in the brain tumor population. The most well described presentation involves dysfunction of the brainstem, either from compression to, or growth within, this region [63, 70, 71]. Tumors that can induce dysphagia in this manner include brainstem glioma, brainstem metastases, ependymoma, choroid plexus papilloma, large pineal region tumors (i.e., pinealoma, astrocytoma), and neoplasms of the cerebellopontine angle such as acoustic schwannoma and meningioma. Direct tumor compression causes impairment of the brainstem circuitry that underlies swallowing, including the nucleus tractus solitarius, ventromedial reticular formation, and cranial nerve motor efferents (V_3, VII, IX, X, XII, and ansa cervicalis) [72–74]. Other reports contend that unilateral, supratentorial tumors can also cause dysphagia [75, 76]. In a prospective analysis of dysphagia in PBT patients and a set of non-brain tumor neurological controls, Newton and colleagues noted that 17 of 117 (14.5%) tumor patients complained of swallowing problems [76]. Formal swallowing assessment of the symptomatic cohort revealed that most patients significantly underestimated their degree of dysfunction. It was also noted that symptomatic patients with decreased level of alertness (LOA) were more likely to have abnormalities during bedside and videofluoroscopic testing. Twelve of the 17 symptomatic patients (70.5%) had large and diffuse, unilateral, supratentorial lesions with surrounding edema and mass effect, often associated with decreased LOA. The neuroanatomical basis for dysphagia from a unilateral lesion remains unclear. However, it is probably due to a combination of several factors, including reduced awareness of oral sensory feedback cues during mastication in patients with reduced LOA, contralateral weakness of the face and tongue, and oral apraxia with impaired motor programming ability for oral-lingual feeding behavior.

Based on the available literature, it would seem prudent to routinely screen all advanced brain tumor patients for dysphagic symptoms, especially in the latter stages of their disease, with or without reduced LOA. All symptomatic patients should undergo a formal swallowing evaluation, even when the complaint seems trivial [76]. The initial bedside screening examination can assess oral and laryngeal function and identify patients at risk for aspiration [77]. In addition, bedside testing can allow modification of eating behavior to diminish the risk of aspiration. Further examination is often needed after the initial bedside evaluation to allow more detailed assessment of the swallowing mechanism, such as delays during the pharyngeal swallow, the degree of laryngeal elevation, pharyngeal symmetry, pooling or coating of pharyngeal recesses, and silent aspiration. The modified barium swallow is used for this assessment and can accurately reveal the abnormalities of the swallowing mechanism, the degree of aspiration, and how best to modify the diet [76, 78, 79].

Management of dysphagic brain tumor patients can often be a complex issue. Patients must be able to demonstrate the necessary cognitive and communication skills to actively participate in a swallowing management program [77, 79]. Tumor patients with diminished LOA or significant cognitive alterations may be unable to pursue complex rehabilitation strategies similar to those used for patients with other neurologic disorders (e.g., stroke). In those patients with adequate LOA, swallowing rehabilitation should be pursued. If compensatory techniques do not improve oral efficiency, an alternate route of nutrition may be required, such as a gastric feeding tube.

Psychiatric Issues

There are several important psychiatric issues that must be assiduously screened for during the care of MBT patients and family members. These issues include depression, associated problems with sleep, and anxiety [80–85]. All cancer patients face numerous stressors during their illness, including fears of a painful death, disability, disfigurement, dependency, and separation from loved ones. The psychological impact of these stressors is quite variable, however, depending on differences in personality, coping mechanisms, social support structure, and medical factors. If cancer patients as a whole are screened using criteria of the Diagnostic and Statistical Manual of Mental Disorders III (DSM III), between 50% and 55% will be shown to have adjusted adequately to the stresses of cancer without exhibiting a diagnosable psychiatric disorder [81]. However, approximately 45% will have a diagnosable psychiatric disorder, of which two thirds will be an adjustment disorder

levels of depression. For most cancer patients with moderate to severe depression, the mainstay of therapy will be pharmacological intervention with an antidepressant medication (see Table 3). There are several classes of antidepressant drugs; comparative clinical trials suggest that the efficacy of drugs within each class and between classes is similar. Clinical improvement usually takes two to three weeks to become evident, with a peak affect at four to six weeks. The first depressive symptoms to improve are mood, quality of sleep, appetite, and personal grooming. Renewed interest in activities and increased energy level occur soon afterwards. In general, depressed cancer patients tend to respond to lower doses of antidepressant medication than patients without cancer. If a patient does not respond to maximal dosing of one antidepressant, a drug from a different class should be attempted next.

Table 3. Antidepressant Drugs Available for Treatment of Depression in Brain Tumor Patients

Drug	Anti-Cholinergic	Sedation	Orthostatic Hypotension	Metabolism	Target Dose (mg/d)
TRICYCLICS					
imipramine	++	++	+++	liver	10–125
amitryptyline	+++	+++	+++	liver	10–125
desipramine	+	+	++	liver	25–125
nortriptyline	++	++	+	liver	25–125
doxepin	++	+++	++	liver	25–125
amoxapine	+	++	+	liver	100–150
protriptyline	+++	+	++	liver	30–60
SELECTIVE SEROTONIN REUPTAKE INHIBITORS					
fluoxetine	+	+	+	liver	20–60
sertraline	0	+	+	liver	50–150
paroxetine	+	+	+	liver	20–50
fluvoxamine	+	+	+	liver	150–200
citalopram	+	+	+	liver	20–60
escitalopram	+	+	+	liver	10–20
OTHER AGENTS					
bupropion	0	0	0	liver	200–400
maprotiline	+	+	++	liver	100–225
amoxapine	+	+	0	liver	200–500
trazodone	++	+++	++	liver	200–600
venlafaxine	+	++	+	liver	75–375
mirtazapine	+	++	+	liver	15–60
nefazodone	+	++	+	liver	300–600

Adapted from references [78–87]
Abbreviations: 0 – negligible, + – mild, ++ – moderate, +++ –severe, mg/d – mg/day

Since antidepressant efficacy is fairly uniform, the choice of drug will mainly depend on the toxicity profile and potential interactions of a given agent in relation to a specific patient and their medical condition [80–82,84]. Depressed patients with agitation, anxiety, and poor sleep would benefit from an antidepressant with sedating effects such as amitriptyline, doxepin, trazodone, nefazodone, or mirtazapine. Patients with depression that manifests psychomotor slowing, fatigue, or sedation from other medications might benefit from an activating antidepressant that causes minimal sedation, such as desipramine or one of the serotonin specific reuptake inhibitors (SSRI's) such as fluoxetine, bupropion, or citalopram. Patients with stomatitis, slowed intestinal motility, or urinary retention should receive an antide-pressant with minimal anticholinergic activity, such as desipramine, nortriptyline, or one of the SSRI's. The tricyclic antidepressants as a class have the potential for cardiotoxicity and should be given with caution to cancer patients with unrelated heart disease. In particular, these drugs should not be prescribed to patients with cardiac conduction abnormalities or bundle-branch block. For the majority of depressed cancer patients, the SSRI's (e.g., fluoxetine, sertraline, paroxetine, fluvoxamine, citalopram) will be the antidepressant drugs of choice [82, 84]. The SSRI's are well tolerated, effective, and associated with less cardiotoxicity and anticholinergic side effects than the tricyclic class of antidepressants. In addition, they are safer in the setting of a depressed cancer patient who attempts suicide by overdose.

Anxiety is common in the cancer patient population, with an incidence of 10% to 30%, and often co-exists with depression [80, 81, 83]. Several anxiety syndromes can be present and include reactive anxiety related to the stress of cancer and its treatment, anxiety that is a manifestation of a medical or physiological problem associated with the cancer (organic anxiety disorder), and pre-morbid phobias or chronic anxiety disorders that are exacerbated by the illness. Reactive anxiety will fluctuate during the course of the patient's illness, becoming more severe during critical moments of bad news. High levels of anxiety can disrupt the patient's ability to function normally, interfere with interpersonal relationships and activities at work, and may impair their ability to comply with cancer therapy. The mainstay of treatment for anxiety is pharmacological therapy with short-acting benzodiazepines such as alprazolam (0.25 to 2.0 mg tid to qid), oxazepam (10 to 15 mg tid to qid), or lorazepam (0.5 to 2.0 mg tid to qid). Patients that experience breakthrough anxiety or end-of-dose failure using a short-acting benzodiazepine may benefit by switching to a longer-acting drug such as diazepam (5 to 10 mg bid to qid) or clonazepam (0.5 to 2.0 mg bid to qid). An alternative drug is the non-benzodiazepine anxiolytic buspirone, which is effective at doses of 5 to 10 mg tid. Neuroleptic drugs such as haloperidol (0.5 to 5 mg bid to qid) or thioridazine (10 to 25 mg tid) may be useful as adjunctive treatment for patients that do not respond well to benzodiazepines or have psychotic features (e.g., hallucinations, delusions) that accompany the anxiety. The most common causes of an organic anxiety disorder in cancer patients are uncon-trolled pain, medication effects (i.e., narcotic analgesics, corticosteroids), infection, and metabolic derangements. Treatment of the underlying medical condition and judicious use of benzodiazepines and/or low-dose antipsychotics are appropriate. In addition to pharmacological approaches, behavioral interventions such as relaxation training, systematic desensitization, and positive imagery techniques can be of benefit to selected patients.

Conclusion

Although the focus of the Treatment Team will be on curative or stabilizing therapy for most patients with MBT, it will still be very important for the treating physician to be aware of the many aspects of supportive care outlined above. Common problems related to seizure control, toxicity of anticonvulsants, prophylaxis and treatment of thromboembolic complications, psychiatric issues, and corticosteroids must be assiduously monitored in every patient.

References

1. Ruhstaller T, Roe H, Thurlimann B, Nicoll JJ. The multidisciplinary meeting: An indispensable aid to communication between different specialties. Eur J Cancer [2006; Epub ahead of print].
2. Ptacek JT, Ptacek JJ. Patients' perceptions of receiving bad news about cancer. J Clin Oncol 2001; 19:4160–4164.
3. Back AL, Arnold RM. Discussing prognosis: "How much do you want to know?" Talking to patients who are prepared for explicit information. J Clin Oncol 2006; 24:4209–4213.
4. Back AL, Arnold RM. Discussing prognosis: "How much do you want to know?" Talking to patients who do not want information or who are ambivalent. J Clin Oncol 2006; 24:4214–4217.
5. Feldman GB. The role of support in treating the brain tumor patient. In: *Cancer of the Nervous System*. Black PM, Loeffler JS (Eds.). Blackwell Science, Cambridge 1997; 17:335–345.
6. Given BA, Given CW, Kozachik S. Family support in advanced cancer. CA Cancer J Clin 2001; 51:213–231.
7. Nijboer C, Tempelaar R, Triemstra M, van den Bos GAM, Sanderman R. The role of social and psychologic resources in caregiving of cancer patients. Cancer 2001; 91:1029–103
8. Glantz M, Recht LD. Epilepsy in the cancer patient. In: *Handbook of Clinical Neurology, Vol. 25 (69): Neuro-Oncology, Part III*. Vecht CJ (Ed.). Elsevier Science, Amsterdam 1997; 2:9–18.
9. Newton HB. Neurological complications of systemic cancer. Amer Fam Phys 1999; 59:878–886.

10. Schaller B, Rüegg SJ. Brain tumor and seizures: Pathophysiology and its implications for treatment revisited. Epilepsia 2003; 44:1223–1232.

11. Ettinger AB. Structural causes of epilepsy: Tumors, cysts, stroke, and vascular malformation. Neurol Clin 1994; 12:41–56.

12. Highland MM, Berger MS, Kunkel DD, Franck JE, Ghatan S, Ojemannn GA. Changes in gamma-aminobutyric acid and somatostatin in epileptic cortex associated with low-grade gliomas. J Neurosurg 1992; 77:209–216.

13. Bateman DE, Hardy JA, McDermott JR, Parker DS, Edwardson JA. Amino acid neurotransmitter levels in gliomas and their relationship to the incidence of epilepsy. Neurol Res 1988; 10:112–114.

14. Ye ZC, Sontheimer H. Glioma cells release excitotoxic concentrations of glutamate. Cancer Res 1999; 59:4383–4391.

15. Behrens PF, Langemann H, Strohschein R, Draeger J, Hennig J. Extracellular glutamate and other metabolites in and around RG2 rat glioma: an intracerebral microdialysis study. J Neuro-Oncol 2000; 47:11–22.

16. Brodie MJ, Dichter MA. Antiepileptic drugs. New Engl J Med 1996; 334: 168–175.

17. Britton JW, So EL. Selection of antiepileptic drugs: A practical approach. Mayo Clin Proc 1996; 71:778–786.

18. Mattson RH, Cramer BS, Collins JF, and the Department of Veterans Affairs Epilepsy Cooperative Study Group. A comparison of valproate with carbamazepine for the treatment of complex partial seizures and secondarily generalized tonic-clonic seizures in adults. New Engl J Med 1992; 327:765–771.

19. Dichter MA, Brodie MJ. New antiepileptic drugs. New Eng J Med 1996; 334:1583–1590.

20. Rosenfeld WE. Topiramate: A review of preclinical, pharmacokinetic, and clinical data. Clin Therap 1997; 19:1294-

21. Newton HB, Goldlust S, Pearl D. Retrospective analysis of the efficacy and tolerability of levetiracetam in brain tumor patients. J Neuro-Oncol 2006; 78:99–102.

22. Vecht CJ, Wagner GL, Wilms EB. Interactions between antiepileptic and chemotherapeutic drugs. Lancet Neurol 2003; 2:404–409.

23. North JB, Penhall RK, Hanieh A, Frewin DB, Taylor WB. Phenytoin and postoperative epilepsy. A double-blind study. J Neurosurg 1983; 58:672–677.

24. Boarini DJ, Beck DW, VanGilder JC. Postoperative prophylactic anticonvulsant therapy in cerebral gliomas. Neurosurg 1985; 16:290–292.

25. Cohen N, Strauss G, Lew R, Silver D, Recht L. Should prophylactic anticonvulsants be administered to patients with newly-diagnosed cerebral metastases? A retrospective analysis. J Clin Oncol 1988; 6:1621–1624.

26. Franceschetti S, Binelli S, Casazza M, et al. Influence of surgery and antiepileptic drugs on seizures symptomatic of cerebral tumours. Acta Neurochir 1990; 103:47–51.

27. Shaw MDM. Post-operative epilepsy and the efficacy of anticonvulsant therapy. Acta Neurochir Suppl 1990; 50:55–57.
28. Foy PM, Chadwick DW, Rajgopalan N, Johnson AL, Shaw MDM. Do prophylactic anticonvulsant drugs alter the pattern of seizures after craniotomy? J Neurol Neurosurg Psych 1992; 55:753–757.
29. Glantz MJ, Cole BF, Friedberg MH, et al. A randomized, blinded, placebo-controlled trial of divalproex sodium prophylaxis in adults with newly diagnosed brain tumors. Neurol 1996; 46:985–991.
30. Glantz MJ, Cole BF, Forsyth PA, et al. Practice parameter: Anticonvulsant prophylaxis in patients with newly diagnosed brain tumors. Report of the Quality Standards Subcommittee of the American Academy of Neurology. Neurol 2000; 54:1886–1893.
31. Newton HB, Turowski RC, Stroup TJ, McCoy LK. Clinical presentation, diagnosis, and pharmacotherapy of patients with primary brain tumors. Ann Pharmacother 1999; 33:816–832.
32. Ohnishi T, Sher PB, Posner JB, Shapiro WB. Capillary permeability factor secreted by malignant brain tumor. Role in peritumoral edema and possible mechanism for anti-edema effect of glucocorticoids. J Neurosurg 1990; 72: 245–251.
33. Del Maestro RF, Megyesi JF, Farrell CL. Mechanisms of tumor-associated edema: A review. Can J Neurol Sci 1990; 17:177–183.
34. Samdani AF, Tamargo RJ, Long DM. Brain tumor edema and the role of the blood-brain barrier, in Vecht CJ (ed.): Handbook of Clinical Neurology, Vol. 23 (67): Neuro-Oncology, Part I. Amsterdam, Elsevier Science, 1997; 4:71–102.
35. Mukwaya G. Immunosuppressive effects and infections associated with corticosteroid therapy. Pediatr Infect Dis J 1988; 7:499–504.
36. Østergaard L, Hochberg FH, Rabinov JD, et al. Early changes measured by magnetic resonance imaging in cerebral blood flow, blood volume, and blood-brain barrier permeability following dexamethasone treatment in patients with brain tumors. J Neurosurg 1999; 90:300–305.
37. Lester RS, Knowles SR, Shear NH. The risks of systemic corticosteroid use. Dermatol Clin 1998; 16:277–286.
38. Weissman DE, Dufer D, Vogel V, Abeloff DD. Corticosteroid toxicity in neuro-oncology patients. J Neuro-Oncol 1987; 5:125–128.
39. Fadul CE, Lemann W, Thaler HT, Posner JB. Perforation of the gastrointestinal tract in patients receiving steroids for neurologic disease. Neurol 1988; 38: 348–352.
40. Stiefel FC, Breitbart WS, Holland JC. Corticosteroids in cancer: Neuropsychiatric complications. Cancer Investig 1989; 7:479–491.
41. Dropcho EJ, Soong SJ. Steroid-induced weakness in patients with primary brain tumors. Neurol 1991; 41:1235–1239.
42. Batchelor TT, Taylor LT, Thaler HT, Posner JB, DeAngelis LM. Steroid myopathy in cancer patients. Neurol 1997; 48:1234–1238.

43. Joseph JC. Corticosteroid-induced osteoporosis. Am J Hosp Pharm 1994; 51:188–197.
44. McIlwain HH. Glucocorticoid-induced osteoporosis: pathogenesis, diagnosis, and management. Preventive Med 2003; 36:243–249.
45. Mahindra AK, Grossman SA. Pneumocystis carinii pneumonia in HIV negative patients with primary brain tumors. J Neuro-Oncol 2003; 63:263–270.
46. Mathew BS, Grossman SA. Pneumocystic carinii pneumonia prophylaxis in HIV negative patients with primary CNS lymphoma. Cancer Treat Rev 2003; 29:105–119.
47. Ellershaw JE, Kelly MJ. Corticosteroids and peptic ulceration. Palliative Med 1994; 8:313–319.
48. Garnett WR, Garabedian-Ruffalo SM. Identification, diagnosis, and treatment of acid-related diseases in the elderly: Implications for long-term care. Pharmacother 1997; 17:938–958.
49. Sachs G. Proton pump inhibitors and acid-related diseases. Pharmacother 1997; 17:22–37.
50. Lee AYY, Levine MN. Management of venous thromboembolism in cancer patients. Oncol 2000; 14:409–421.
51. Gomes MPV, Deitcher SR. Diagnosis of venous thromboembolic disease in cancer patients. Oncol 2003; 17:126–139.
52. Sawaya R, Zuccarello M, Elkalliny M, Nighiyama H. Postoperative venous thromboembolism and brain tumors: part I. Clinical profile. J Neuro-Oncol 1992; 14:119–125.
53. Hamilton MG, Hull RD, Pineo GF. Venous thromboembolism in neurosurgery and neurology patients: A review. Neurosurg 1994; 34:280–296.
54. Marras LC, Geerts WH, Perry JR. The risk of venous thromboembolism is increased throughout the course of malignant glioma. An evidence-based review. Cancer 2000; 89:640–646.
55. Brandes AA, Scelzi E, Salmistraro E, et al. Incidence and risk of thromboembolism during treatment of high-grade gliomas: a prospective study. Eur J Cancer 1997; 33:1592–1596.
56. Quevedo JF, Buckner JC, Schmidt JL, Dinapoli RP, O'Fallon JR. Thromboembolism in patients with high-grade glioma. Mayo Clin Proc 1994; 69:329–332.
57. Ruff RL, Posner JB. The incidence and treatment of peripheral venous thrombosis in patients with glioma. Ann Neurol 1983; 13:334–336.
58. Altshuler E, Moosa H, Selker RG, Vertosick FT. The risk and efficacy of anticoagulant therapy in the treatment of thromboembolic complications in patients with primary brain tumors. Neurosurg 1990; 27:74–77.
59. Levin JM, Schiff D, Loeffler JS, Fine HA, Black PML, Wen PY. Complications of therapy for venous thromboembolic disease in patients with brain tumors. Neurol 1993; 43:1111–1114.
60. Schiff D, DeAngelis LM. Therapy of venous thromboembolism in patients with brain metastases. Cancer 1994; 73:493–498.

61. Weitz JI. Low-molecular-weight heparins. New Engl J Med 1997; 337: 688–698.
62. Dorfman GS. Evaluating the roles and functions of vena caval filters: will data be available before or after these devices are removed from the market? Radiol 1992; 185:15–17.
63. Buchholz D. Neurologic causes of dysphagia. Dysphagia 1987; 1:152–156.
64. Kirshner HS. Causes of Neurogenic dysphagia. Dysphagia 1989; 3:184–188.
65. Barer DH. The natural history and functional consequences of dysphagia after hemispheric stroke. J Neurol Neurosurg Psychiatry 1989; 52:236–241.
66. Lieberman AN, Horowitz L, Redmond P, Pachter L, Lieberman I, Leibowitz M. Dysphagia in Parkinson's disease. Am J Gastroenterol 1980; 74:157–160.
67. Daly DD, Code CF, Anderson HA. Disturbances of swallowing and esophageal motility in patients with multiple sclerosis. Neurol 1962; 59:250–256.
68. Robbins J. Swallowing in ALS and motor neuron disease. Neurol Clin 1987; 5:213–229
69. Buchholz D. Neurologic evaluation of dysphagia. Dysphagia 1987; 1:187–192.
70. Frank Y, Schwartz SB, Epstein NE, Beresford HR. Chronic dysphagia, vomiting and gastroesophageal reflux as manifestations of a brain stem glioma: A case report. Pediatr Neurosci 1989; 15:265–268.
71. Straube A, Witt TN. Oculo-bulbar myasthenic symptoms as the sole sign of tumour involving or compressing the brain stem. J Neurol 1990; 237:369–371.
72. Cunningham ET, Donner MW, Jones B, Point SM. Anatomical and physiological overview, in Jones B, Donner MW (Eds.): *Normal and Abnormal Swallowing. Imaging in Diagnosis and Therapy.* Springer-Verlag, New York, 1991; 2:7–32.
73. Dodds WJ, Stewart ET, Logemann JA. Physiology and radiology of the normal oral and pharyngeal phases of swallowing. Am J Roentgenol 1989; 154: 953–963.
74. Sessle BJ, Henry JL. Neural mechanisms of swallowing: Neurophysiological and neurochemical studies on brain stem neurons in the solitary tract region. Dysphagia 1989; 4:61–75.
75. Meadows JC. Dysphagia in unilateral cerebral lesions. J Neurol Neurosurg Psych 1973; 36:853–860.
76. Newton HB, Newton C, Pearl D, Davidson T. Swallowing assessment in primary brain tumor patients with dysphagia. Neurol 1994; 44:1927–1932.
77. Emick-Herring B, Wood P. A team approach to neurologically based swallowing disorders. Rehabil Nurs 1990; 15:126–132.
78. Dodds WJ, Logemann JA, Stewart ET. Radiologic assessment of abnormal oral and pharyngeal phases of swallowing. Am J Roentgenol 1990; 154:965–974.
79. Bloch AS. Nutritional management of patients with dysphagia. Oncol 1993; 7:127–137.
80. Levine SH, Jones LD, Sack DA. Evaluation and treatment of depression, anxiety, and insomnia in patients with cancer. Oncol 1993; 7:119–125.

81. Breitbart W. Psycho-Oncology: Depression, anxiety, delirium. Sem Oncol 1994; 21:754–769.
82. Pirl WF, Roth AJ. Diagnosis and treatment of depression in cancer patients. Oncol 1999; 13:1293–1301.
83. Stark D, Kiely M, Smith A, Vilikova G, House A, Selby P. Anxiety disorders in cancer patients: Their nature, associations, and relation to quality of life. J Clin Oncol 2002; 20:3137–3148.
84. Schwartz L, Lander M, Chochinov HM. Current management of depression in cancer patients. Oncol 2002; 16:1102–1110.
85. Maguire P. Improving the recognition of concerns and affective disorders in cancer patients. Ann Oncol 2002; 13:177–181.
86. American Psychiatric Association: *Diagnostic and Statistical Manual of Mental Disorders*, 4th ed. Washington, DC. American Psychiatric Association, 1994; 317–391.
87. Bukberg J, Penman D, Holland JC. Depression in hospitalized cancer patients. Psychosomatics 1984; 46:199–212.
88. Redd WH, Montgomery GH, DuHamel KN. Behavioral intervention for cancer treatment side effects. J Natl Cancer Inst 2001; 93:810–823.
89. Newell SA, Sanson-Fisher RW, Savolainen NJ. Systematic review of psychological therapies for cancer patients: Overview and recommendations for future research. J Natl Cancer Inst 2002; 94:558–584.

increased success of the neuro-oncology team in controlling intracranial disease, more patients are succumbing to progressive extracranial disease [5]. Therefore, to maximize quality of life, it is critical to minimize the morbidity associated with surgery. The factors relevant in predicting the occurrence of postoperative morbidity, particularly neurological deficit, are the location of the lesion within the brain and the surgical corridor required to reach it. Morbidity incurred during creation of the surgical corridor includes not only the iatrogenic injury to the overlying brain a surgeon must traverse to reach the lesion below the brain surface, but also the extent of secondary injury that can be caused by brain manipulation and retraction during the surgical resection. These factors must temper the surgeon's overall approach, and demand judicious use of accessory technologies to increase the safety of surgery.

The care of patients with brain metastases requires a multidisciplinary approach; during surgery, the anesthesiologist is an equal partner in the maintenance of the patient's well-being. Constant communication between the surgeon and the anesthesiologist results in a seamless procedure that begins with the administration of parenteral antibiotics for prevention of surgery-related wound infections, dexamethasone for reduction of brain edema, and often mannitol or a supplementary diuretic to achieve reduced brain tension [23, 24]. Aggressive hyperventilation is not required: an arterial $PaCO2$ of 32 to 37 mmHg is adequate. At the time of surgery, a therapeutic serum level of an anticonvulsant should be attained and is maintained for one week after surgery [25]; the use of AEDs is discussed in more detail later in this chapter.

On the morning of surgery, patients undergo a contrast-enhanced stereotactic magnetic resonance imaging (MRI) study of the brain. After the patient is positioned on the operating room table, general endotracheal anesthesia is induced, and the patient's head is affixed to the operating table with a three-point head holder. The fiducials on the patient are registered with the stereotactic surgical navigation device and the target is precisely localized, the appropriate trajectory to the tumor is selected, and a tailored incision is designed [26, 27]. This presurgical planning is an important step to ensure success. Image-based planning is used to identify the shortest route to the tumor through noneloquent brain, which requires the microsurgical dissection of a sulcus, but the effort is rewarded by the creation of a corridor to the tumor that results in the least disruption of cortex.

Large tumors are often debulked from within utilizing the ultrasonic aspirator to minimize the risk of incurring neurological morbidity due to tissue manipulation and placement of brain retraction devices (Figure 1). Once the bulk of the tumor has been reduced from within, the dissection of the tumor proceeds by folding the tumor in on itself, again minimizing the retraction on the surrounding brain parenchyma. All vessels in the vicinity of the tumor are confirmed to enter the tumor before bipolar coagulation; this ensures that the blood supply to the adjacent normal brain is not compromised. After achieving complete dissection from the normal brain, the tumor

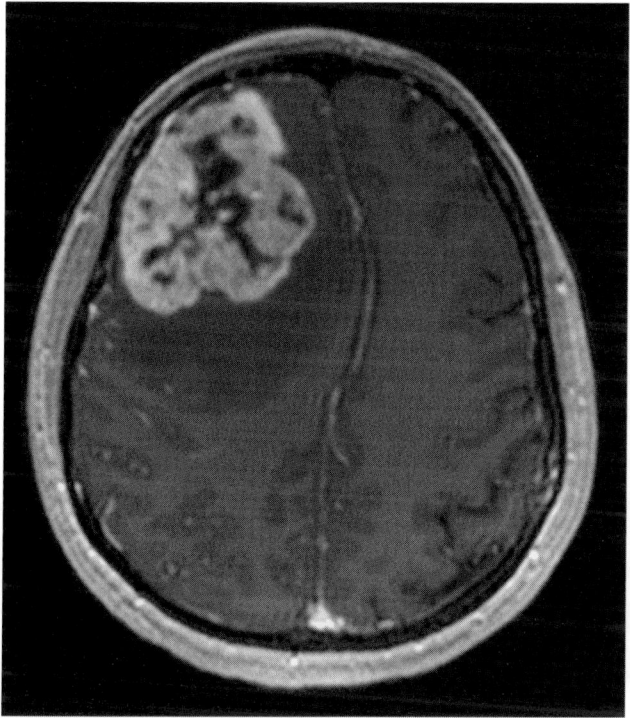

Figure 1. A large right frontal solitary metastasis in a patient with a history of breast cancer diagnosed three years prior to presentation. Note the mass effect, midline shift, and the brain edema.

is removed from the surgical bed. Extra time spent ensuring adequate hemostasis is a vital step to avoid a postoperative complication such as an operative site hematoma.

Careful closure of the craniotomy is an equally important step to avoid postoperative complications, namely the risk of a cerebrospinal fluid leak, which dramatically increases the risk of an infection. A water-tight dural closure is accomplished, followed by securing of the craniotomy bone flap to the skull. The fascia overlying the muscle layer is then reapproximated and the scalp closed in two layers. It is rare to require the placement of a surgical site closed-suctioning drainage tube in elective craniotomies.

Special Anatomic Considerations:

Approaches to deep-seated lesions in areas such as the thalamus (Figure 2) and brainstem are associated with unacceptable risks, usually resulting in iatrogenic injury to cortical and subcortical structures and navigation in limited surgical ventricular catheter is placed following induction of general anesthesia but prior to craniotomy, to facilitate brain relaxation and prevent herniation during the dural opening. Another special consideration with cerebellar lesions is that, in contrast to lesions in the supratentorial compartment, AEDs are not utilized metastases due to the very rare occurrence of seizures [28].

The Role of Technology in Surgery

A key technological "assistant" for the neurosurgeon is the stereotactic surgical navigation device, which allows the surgeon to localize the lesion and design the incision before the actual operation ensues. Device set-up adds minimal time to the preoperative preparation, and is more than accounted for by the benefits derived in terms of the intra-operative localization of the lesion, choice of sulcal dissection, and trajectory of approach through the cortex.

When stereotaxy is not employed, the surgeon must rely on the patient's surface landmarks for preoperative lesion localization and design of the craniotomy. Usually, a larger craniotomy is made in these situations compared to that made in a stereotaxis-guided approach to compensate for any errors in lesion localization, although in experienced hands, the lesion is usually located within a centimeter or two of the surgeon's estimate. Once the craniotomy has been performed and the dura mater incised, the cortical surface should be inspected for any signs of an underlying metastatic lesion, such as gyral expansion or increased vascularity. It is not common for a metastatic lesion to come to the pial surface or to have dural representation (Figure 5); in those cases, the intra-operative ultrasonography may help to locate the metastatic lesion, which is often echogenic in nature. Cystic lesions are easily differentiated from the surrounding parenchyma and depending on the location of the lesion, the patient's normal anatomic landmarks such as the falx cerebri or the ventricular system may be used as further localizing structures [29].

During surgery in or adjacent to eloquent cortical areas, the use of electro-corticography and awake craniotomy may reduce the surgical risk by identi-fying eloquent cortical and subcortical areas [30]. With intraoperative stimulation mapping, a constant-current generator is used to deliver biphasic square-wave pulses to depolarize cortical neurons or their pathways in the white matter. Motor or language areas can be delineated by electrocorticography performed while asking an awake patient to complete a motor or linguistic task. The expertise of the anesthesia

Figure 4. Intra-operative photograph of the tumor bed in Figure 3 after resection, demon-strating the preservation of all the superficial cortical veins, which were draped over the tumor mass. Injury to these veins could result in a venous infarction, with severe conse-quences. Note the minimal amount of normal brain exposed during this stereotaxis-guided surgery.

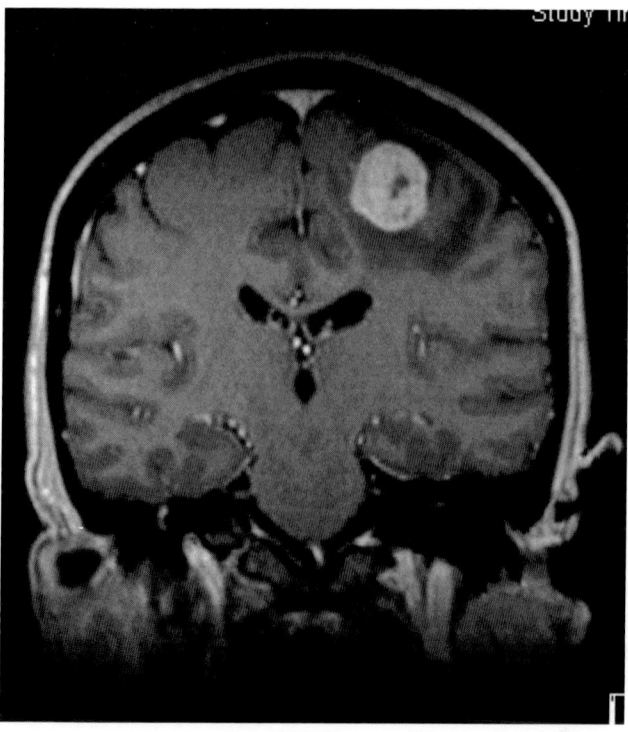

Figure 5. The typical location for metastatic lesions – within the substance of the brain, with the epicenter in the region of the gray-white matter junction, with no pial representation.

staff is of utmost importance during intra-operative testing procedures, as a balance in extent of anesthesia must be achieved to allow the patient to remain comfortable, yet still be able to participate with the surgical team. Awake craniotomy is often very well tolerated, although its consideration does require a careful preoperative assessment of the patient's capacity to cooperate and participate with testing.

Medical Postoperative Care

Antiepileptic Drugs (AED)

It is well appreciated that AEDs may have potentially severe, even life-threatening, side effects, and should be used judiciously [25]. In a recent position paper, the American Academy of Neurology (AAN) recommended that patients undergoing surgery for intracranial metastatic disease without a history of prior seizure be treated with dexamethasone and an AED in the perioperative period, but that the AED agent should be tapered after one week [31]. In patients who present with

2. Posner JP. Management of brain metastases. Rev Neurol (Paris) 1992; 148: 477–487.
3. Nusbaum ES, Djalilian HR, Cho KH, et al. Brain metastases: histology, multiplicity, surgery, and survival. Cancer 1996; 78: 1781–1788.
4. Salvati M, Cervoni L, Raco A. Single brain metastases from unknown primary malignancies in CT-era. J Neurooncol 1995; 23:75–80.
5. Patchell RA, Tibbs PA, Walsh JW et al. A randomized trial of surgery in the treatment of single brain metastases to the brain: A randomized trial. N Eng J Med 1990; 322:494–500.
6. Peacock KH, Lesser GJ. Current therapeutic approaches in patients with brain metastases. Curr Treat Options Oncol 2006; 7:479–489.
7. Bindal RK, Sawaya R, Leavens ME et al. Surgical treatment of multiple brain metastases. J Neurosurg 1993; 79:210–216.
8. Brega K, Robinson WA, Winston K et al. Surgical treatment of brain metastases in malignant melanoma. Cancer 1990; 66:2105–2110.
9. Sundaresan N, Galicich JH. Surgical treatment of brain metastases. Clinical and computerized tomography evaluation of the results of treatment. Cancer 1985; 55:1382–1388.
10. Constantini S, Kornowski R, Pomeranz S et al. Thromboembolic phenomena in neurosurgical patients operated upon for primary and metastatic brain tumors. Acta Neurochir (Wien). 1991; 109:93–97.
11. Sawaya R, Donlon JA. Chronic disseminated intravascular coagulation and metastatic brain tumor: a case report and review of the literature. Neurosurg 1983;12:580–584.
12. Gaspar L, Scott C, Rotman M et al. Recursive partitioning analysis (RPA) of prognostic factors in three Radiation Therapy Oncology Group (RTOG) brain metastases trials. In J Radiat Oncol Biol Phys 1997; 37:745–751.
13. Morris SL, Low SH, A'Hern RP, et al. A prognostic index that predicts outcome following palliative whole brain radiotherapy for patient with metastatic melanoma. Br J Cancer 2004; 91: 829–33.
14. Vecht CJ, Haaxma-Reiche H, Noordijk EM et al. Treatment of single brain metastases: radiotherapy alone or combined with neurosurgery? Ann Neurol 1993; 33:583–590.
15. Mintz AH, Kestle J, Rathbone MP, et al. A randomized trial to assess the efficacy of surgery in addition to radiotherapy in patients with a single cerebral metastasis. Cancer 1996; 78:1470–1476.
16. Wronski M, Arbit E. Resection of brain metastases from colorectal carcinoma in 73 patients. Cancer. 1999; 85:1677–1685.
17. Iwadate Y, Namba H, Yamaura A. Significance of surgical resection for the treatment of multiple brain metastases. Anticancer Res 2000; 20: 573–7.
18. Pollock BE, Brown PD, Foote RL, et al. Properly selected patients with multiple brain metastases may benefit from aggressive treatment of their intracranial disease. J Neurooncol 2003; 61: 73–80.

19. Schackert G, Steinmetz A, Meier U, et al. Surgical management of single and multiple brain metastases: results of a retrospective study. Onkologie 2001; 24Ú 246–55.

20. Weber F, Riedel A, Koning W, et al. The role of adjuvant radiation and multiple resection within the surgical management of brain metastases. Neurosurg Rev 1996; 19: 23–32.

21. Nieder C, Andratschke N, Grosu AL et al. Recursive partitioning analysis (RPA) class does not predict survival in patients with four or more brain metastases. Strahlenther Onkol 2003; 179:16–20.

22. Arbit E, Wronski M, Burt M, Galicich JH. The treatment of patient s with recurrent brain metastases. A retrospective analysis of 109 patients with nonsmall cell lung cancer. Cancer 1995; 76: 765–73.

23. Barker FG. Efficacy of prophylactic antibiotics for craniotomy: A meta-analysis. Neurosurgery 1994; 35: 484–92.

24. Galicich JH and French LA. Use of dexamethasone in the treatment of cerebral edema resulting from brain tumors and brain surgery. Am Pract Dig Treat 1961; 12: 169–74.

25. Shaw MD and Foy PM. Epilepsy after craniotomy and the place of prophylactic anticonvulsant drugs: discussion paper. J R Soc Med 1991; 84: 221–223.

26. Kondziolka D and Lunsford LD. Intraoperative navigation during resection of brain metastases. Neurosurg Clin N Am 1996; 7: 267–77.

27. Tan TC and Black PM. Image-guided craniotomy for cerebral metastases: techniques and outcomes. Neurosurgery 2003; 53: 82–89.

28. Cohen N, Strauss G, Lew R et al. Should prophylactic anticonvulsants be administered to patients with newly diagnosed cerebral metastases? A retrospective study. J Clin Oncol 1988; 6: 1621–24.

29. Regelsberger J, Lohmann F, Helmke K, et al. Ultrasound-guided surgery of deep seated brain lesions. European Journal of Ultrasound 2000; 12: 115–21.

30. Keles GE, Lundin DA, Lamborn, KR, et al. Intraoperative subcortical stimulation mapping for hemispheric perirolandic gliomas located within or adjacent to the descending motor pathways: evaluation of morbidity and assessment of functional outcome in 294 patients. J Neurosurg 2004; 100: 369–75.

31. Glantz MJ, Cole BF, Forsyth PA, et al. Practice parameter: Anticonvulsant prophylaxis in patients with newly diagnosed brain tumors. Neurology 2000; 54: 1886–93.

32. Hamilton MG, Hull RD, and Pineo GF. Venous thromboembolism in neurosurgery and neurology patients: A review. Neurosurgery 1994; 34: 280–96.

33. Agnelli G, Piovella F, Buoncristiani P, et al. Enoxaparin plus compression stockings compared with compression stockings alone in the prevention of venous thromboembolism after elective neurosurgery. N Engl J Med 1993; 339: 80–85.

34. Black PM, Baker MF, and Snook CP. Experience with external pneumatic calf compression in neurology and neurosurgery. Neurosurgery 1986; 18: 440–44.

35. Frim DM, Barker FG, Poletti CE, et al. Postoperative low-dose heparin decreases thromboembolic complications in neurosurgical patients. Neurosurgery 1992; 30: 830–33.
36. Danish SF, Burnett MG, Ong JG, et al. Prophylaxis for deep venous thrombosis in craniotomy patients: A decision analysis. Neurosurgery 2005; 56: 1286–1294.
37. Westphal M, Hilt DC, Bortey E, et al. A phase 3 trial of local chemotherapy with biodegradable carmustine (BCNU) wafers (Gliadel wafers) in patients with primary malignant glioma. Neuro-Oncology 2003; 5: 79–88.
38. Brem S, Staller A, and Wotoczek-Obadia Mea. Interstitial chemotherapy for local control of CNS metastases. Presented at the annual meeting of the Society of Neuro-Oncology, Toronto, ON, Canada, November 18–21, 2004 (abstr TA-06).
39. Rogers LR, Rock JP, Sills AK, et al. Results of a phase II trial of the GliaSite radiation therapy system for the treatment of newly diagnosed, resected single brain metastases. J Neurosurg 2006; 105: 375–84.
40. Bobo RH, Laske DW, Akbasak A, et al. Convection-enhanced delivery of macromolecules in the brain. Proc. Natl. Acad. Sci. 1994; 91: 2076–80.
41. Muro K, Das S, Raizer, J. Convection-enhanced delivery of targeted cytotoxins to the central nervous system. Technology in Cancer Research and Treatment 2006; 5: 201–13.
42. Grossi PM, Ochiai II, Archer GE, et al. Efficacy of intracerebral microinfusion of trastuzumab in an athymic rat model of intracerebral metastatic breast cancer. Clin Cancer Res 2003; 9: 5514–20.

6. Radiation for Brain Metastases

Malika L. Siker, M.D. and Minesh P. Mehta, M.D.

Keywords: brain metastases, radiation, radiosurgery, neurocognitive function, motexafin gadolinium, efaproxiril, temozolomide

Introduction

The use of radiotherapy in the treatment of brain metastases includes whole brain radiotherapy (WBRT), either as definitive or as adjuvant treatment following resection or radiosurgery, radiosurgery alone, and brachytherapy. WBRT has been the primary treatment for brain metastases for over 50 years, improving local control and survival as well as providing effective palliation. While definitive WBRT remains the standard of care for most patients, adjuvant WBRT with radiosurgery and surgical resection has been shown to improve local control and survival in a subset of patients [1–3]. The optimal combination of WBRT, radiosurgery, and resection remains to be elucidated, including appropriate timing or sequence.

The goals of treatment are to provide symptomatic relief, improve neurologic status, and prolong survival while taking into account the toxicities of radiotherapy. Neurocognitive impairment, which may be related to the tumor itself, surgery, and/or systemic agents, is one of the potential sequelae of radiotherapy. Managing and preventing neurocognitive impairment is a key issue in radiotherapy for brain metastases.

Systemic agents may have a synergistic effect when used in conjunction with radiotherapy in patients with brain metastases. Chemotherapeutic agents such as temozolomide and radiosensitizers such as motexafin gadolinium (MGd) have shown promising results in clinical trials, when combined with WBRT. Despite these advances beyond WBRT, median survival time has remained fixed at around 4 to 6 months as shown in randomized trials. Optimizing the multimodality approach to improve local control, survival, neurocognitive function, and palliation is the subject of active research. Further clinical trials are needed to provide more refined treatment guidelines.

This chapter will review the role of radiotherapy in the treatment of brain metastases using an evidence-based approach, discussing the use of WBRT and focal treatments. The importance of neurocognitive function and emerging chemical modifiers will be discussed. Treatment recommendations will be provided.

Definitive WBRT

One of the earliest reviews of the use of WBRT appeared in 1954; Chao et al. found that 63% of patients with brain metastases had relief of symptoms and proposed the optimal dose at 30 Gy [4]. Prior to the use of WBRT, survival of patients with brain metastases was a dismal 1–2 months from diagnosis [5, 6]. Over the last 3 decades, a number of randomized trials in the treatment of brain metastases have demonstrated improved local or locoregional control and an increased median survival time of around 4–6 months with WBRT [7, 8]. The appropriate use of WBRT can provide rapid attenuation of many neurologic symptoms, improve quality of life, and is especially beneficial in patients with large, multiple, or diffuse metastases, patients whose lesions impinge on eloquent areas, and patients with medical comorbidities which preclude them from surgery. Multiple metastases (more than one) are found in approximately 80% of patients with brain metastases, making definitive WBRT the treatment of choice for the majority of patients [9].

According to some reports, 60% of patients achieve a complete (CR) or partial (PR) response to WBRT, but these are pre-MR data that have not been adequately validated. Response may depend on histology. CT-determined response rates (CR plus PR) to WBRT for small cell lung cancer (81%) and breast cancer (65%) have been found to be superior to those for renal cell carcinoma (46%) and melanoma (0%) based on an institutional analysis of 108 patients [10]. In a retrospective study of breast cancer patients, 116 women had a median survival of 4.2 months after WBRT alone [11]. In a retrospective study of 74 patients with malignant melanoma, subjects treated with WBRT alone had a median survival of 2.3 month [12]. However, It has been reported that for recurrent brain metastases outcome is not affected by tumor histology [13].

Regardless of histology, actuarial local control at one year after WBRT alone has been found to be 0–14% in randomized trials suggesting that long-term control of brain metastases following conventional treatment is achieved in only a minority [14, 15]. The majority of patients who are locally controlled die of extracranial disease, while patients with recurrent brain metastases typically succumb to central nervous system (CNS) disease [13].

Pretreatment characteristics have been found to be the best predictors of outcome. Recursive partitioning analysis (RPA), a statistical tool that stratifies patients into prognostic groups based on pretreatment patient and tumor characteristics yields a useful prognostic classification. Using RPA, the Radiation Therapy Oncology Group (RTOG) has identified a 3-tiered prognostic classification shown in Table 1

Table 1. Recursive partitioning analysis classes for brain metastases

	Characteristics	MOS
Class I	KPS ≥ 70, primary tumor controlled, age < 65 years, metastases in brain only	7.1 months
Class II	KPS ≥ 70, primary tumor uncontrolled, age ≥ 65 years, metastases in brain and other sites	4.2 months
Class III	KPS < 70	2.3 months

MOS, median overall survival; KPS, Karnofsky performance status.
SOURCE: Data from Gaspar et al. [8]

[8, 16]. Favorable prognostic factors include good performance status, control of the primary tumor, age less than 65 years, and metastases located in the brain only [8]. Patients in RPA class 1 have the longest median survival following WBRT, while patients in RPA class 2 and 3 survive for significantly shorter time periods.

Dose and Schedule

Several different dose, timing, and fractionation schema have been investigated in randomized trials by the RTOG; however, none of these trials have demonstrated superior survival compared to conventional treatment (Table 2) [7,17–23]. Furthermore, accelerated hyperfractionated schedules have not shown any benefit compared to standard treatment in phase III trials [23–25]. Although the optimal schedule is still debated, typical WBRT regimens given in the United States for the treatment of brain metastases include 10 fractions of 3 Gy (30 Gy) over 2 weeks or 15 fractions of 2.5 Gy (37.5 Gy) over 3 weeks. Because of the potential for increased risk of neurocognitive impairment in patients with prolonged survival, some clinicians prefer using schedules that employ prolonged administration times,

Table 2. Randomized trials evaluating different WBRT fractionation regimens

Study	n	Treatment (Gy/number of fractions)	MOS (months)
Harwood et al. [17]	101	30/10 vs. 10/1	4.0 – 4.3
Borgelt et al. [7]	138	10/1 vs. 30/10 vs. 40/20	4.2 – 4.8
Kurtz et al. [18]	255	30/10 vs. 50/20	3.9 – 4.2
Borgelt et al. [19]	64	12/2 vs. 20/5	2.8 – 3.0
Chatani et al. [20]	70	30/10 vs. 50/20	3.0 – 4.0
Haie-Meder et al. [21]	216	18/3 vs. 36/6 vs. 43/13	4.2 – 5.3
Chatani et al. [22]	72	30/10 vs. 50/20 vs. 20/5	2.4 – 4.3
Murray et al. [23]	445	54.4/34 vs. 30/10	4.5

N, number; MOS, months.

such as 3 to 4 weeks, with a simultaneous reduction in dose per fraction for patients with better prognoses. This approach has not yet been validated in prospective, randomized clinical studies.

Complications

Complications of WBRT can be acute or delayed. Acute toxicities, appearing less than 90 days after treatment, associated with WBRT include alopecia, dermatitis, otitis externa, otitis media, hearing loss, nausea or vomiting, and somnolence. Most of these resolve relatively soon after the cessation of treatment. Late toxicities, occurring more than 90 days after treatment, may involve necrosis, personality changes, memory loss, cerebellar dysfunction, cataracts, and neurocognitive deterioration.

In addition to the toxicities of WBRT, some have suggested that the survival is too short and meaningful palliation is not achieved by enough patients to justify WBRT in all patients, although these data are relatively sparse and not reproduced by others [26]. Nevertheless, when balancing the potential benefits of symptomatic relief, improvement in neurologic status, and increased survival with limited toxicities (especially with proper dosage and modern fractionation schemes) and poor outcome without definitive treatment, WBRT remains the standard of care for patients with multiple brain metastases.

WBRT with Focal Treatment

With overall survival fixed at 4 to 6 months despite attempts to improve WBRT delivery, combining WBRT with focal treatment such as resection or radiosurgery has emerged as another approach for these patients. Focal treatment combined with WBRT has been shown to improve overall survival in patients with a single metastasis based on the results of prospective randomized trials. The use of these modalities in combination with WBRT in patients with more than 1 metastasis has not been defined.

Resection and WBRT

With improved surgical technique and post-operative care developed in the 1990s resulting in a decline in mortality to less than 5%, surgery has made a significant contribution in the management of brain metastases [2]. Surgery is indicated when tissue is needed via craniotomy or stereotactic biopsy to establish diagnosis and for resection in patients where tumor removal will provide immediate palliation. Resection followed by WBRT has been shown to significantly improve survival in patients with a single brain metastasis in 2 prospective randomized controlled studies, providing level 1 evidence to justify this method as standard care in these patients [2, 3]. A third phase III trial was unable to reproduce these results, but this trial has been criticized due to the high proportion of patients with poor performance status and extracranial disease as compared to the former trials [27]. These trials suggest that the benefit may be greatest in patients with stable disease, minimal systemic dissemination, younger age, and good performance status. The results of these trials are reviewed in Table 3. Although some preliminary data suggest that resection may increase survival in patients with more than one brain metastasis, this approach has not been validated in a prospective randomized trial [28]. This topic is discussed in more detail in Chapter 5, Surgery for Brain Metastases.

Radiosurgery and WBRT

Stereotactic radiosurgery is a technique that delivers precise, conformal radiation to a defined target in a single large dose. The use of multiple convergent beams allows for sparing of the maximum amount of surrounding normal tissue with rapid dose fall-off at the edge of the target volume. Radiosurgery may be delivered using gamma rays via a Gamma Knife, x-rays by a linear accelerator, or charged particles such as protons using a cyclotron. It is primarily used to treat small lesions (less than 3 cm) in eloquent areas and residual disease after surgical resection. It is minimally invasive and well-tolerated by patients who are not surgical candidates. It is best suited for patients with good performance status and limited extra-cranial disease [29]. Potential adverse effects include swelling, nausea, dizziness, seizures, and headache. Radionecrosis may appear in approximately 5% of patients [30, 31]. In patients with brain metastases, local control rates range from 25–100% with a mean of 81% and response rates vary from 30–100% with an average of 69% [32–34].

Maximum tolerated doses for radiosurgery in the treatment of brain metastases were established in a prospective trial from the RTOG [30]. In this dose-escalation trial, 156 patients, 100 of whom had recurrent brain metastases (64%), underwent

Table 3. Prospective studies of surgery plus WBRT vs. WBRT alone in patients with a single brain metastasis

Study	Treatment	n	MOS	P	FI (weeks)
Patchell et al. [2]	Surgery + WBRT 36 Gy vs.	25	40 weeks	< 0.1	38
	WBRT 36 Gy	23	15 weeks		8
Noordjik et al. [3]	Surgery + WBRT 40 Gy vs.	32	10 months	0.04	33
	WBRT 40 Gy	31	6 months		15
Mintz et al. [27]	Surgery + WBRT 30 Gy vs.	41	5.6 months	0.24	9
	WBRT 30 Gy	43	6.3 months		8

WBRT, whole brain radiation therapy; n, number of patients; MOS, median overall survival; FI, functional independence.

dose escalation in 3 Gy increments until unacceptable toxicity was reached. Investigators were unwilling to continue dose escalation to 27 Gy. The maximum tolerated doses (deemed maximum, without actually reaching toxicity in the smallest diameter group) were 24, 18, and 15 Gy, for tumors less than 20, 21–20, and 31–40 mm, respectively, in maximum diameter.

The first two prospective randomized trials examining the use of radiosurgery with WBRT versus WBRT alone in patients with brain metastases demonstrated enhanced local control in the radiosurgery arm; however these trials have been criticized for poor design [15, 35]. The largest and most recent trial by Andrews et al. confirmed these findings and showed superior survival in patients with a single metastasis treated with WBRT and radiosurgery [1]. In this multi-institutional RTOG trial, 333 patients with 1–3 brain metastases were randomized to receive WBRT alone to 37.5 Gy in 15 fractions (n = 164) or WBRT followed by radiosurgery (n = 167). Although there was no significant improvement in overall survival between the 2 arms (6.5 vs. 5.7 months, p = 0.13), patients with a single brain metastasis (a pre-specified subgroup at the time of trial design for separate analysis from the 2–3 brain metastases cohort) demonstrated a survival advantage when treated with WBRT plus radiosurgery compared to radiosurgery (6.5 vs. 4.9 months, p = 0.04). At 6 months follow-up, patients in the radiosurgery arm were more likely to have stable or improved performance status (43% vs. 37%, p = 0.03). Results from this trial provide level 1 evidence supporting the use of radiosurgery in patients with a single metastasis.

Additionally, a multi-institutional retrospective review suggests that WBRT with radiosurgery may improve survival in patients with brain metastases in all 3 RTOG RPA classes [36]. Five hundred and two patients were stratified by RPA class and survival was calculated using Kaplan-Meier estimates. The addition of radiosurgery to WBRT resulted in improved survival in all 3 RPA classes. A higher performance status, controlled primary, absence of extracranial metastases, and lower RPA predicted for improved survival suggesting that these patients with these characteristics may benefit the most from radiosurgery.

Based on these trials, there is level 1 evidence to support the use of radiosurgery as a boost to WBRT in patients with a single brain metastasis to maximize local control and survival. The role of radiosurgery and WBRT in patients with more than one brain metastasis has yet to be defined, as radiosurgery in these patients improves local control without a significant survival benefit. Retrospective trials suggest that certain patients with multiple metastases may benefit from the addition of radiosurgery; however, this approach cannot be recommended as standard of care at this time [37].

Resection vs. Radiosurgery

A prospective study directly comparing resection and radiosurgery has not been completed. At the 2005 International Stereotactic Radiosurgery Society, Muacevic et al. presented the results of a trial that attempted to further define this question. In this study, 70 patients were randomized to WBRT plus resection or radiosurgery alone. Survival was found to be equivalent in both arms; however the trial was closed due to poor accrual with only 29% of patients accrued. Comparison of functional independence in reports examining radiosurgery or resection with WBRT suggests that treatment with radiosurgery and WBRT results in comparable outcome. Data from retrospective single institution studies directly comparing the outcomes of both modalities have reported conflicting results and are of limited value due to the inherent selection bias found in this type of study [38, 39]. Since there has never been a prospective randomized direct comparison of resection and radiosurgery, a definitive conclusion regarding this question is not possible at this time.

In the absence of level 1 evidence, the decision to use resection or radiosurgery in patients with a single brain metastasis should consider patient and tumor characteristics such as medical co-morbidities that may influence the ability of the patient to tolerate resection, functional status, as well as the location and size of the intracranial lesion. Radiosurgery offers an alternative to resection and may be especially useful in patients who have a single lesion that impinges on an eloquent area or those who are unable to tolerate surgery. Additionally, radiosurgery has been found to be more cost-effective compared to resection [40]. Resection may be preferred when the diagnosis is in doubt, when immediate relief of major increase in intracranial pressure is necessary, and when the lesion is large (greater than 3–4 cm). For all patients, a team approach weighing the advantages and disadvantages of both options is recommended.

Focal Treatment Alone

With the increased efficacy of focal treatments, the use of resection or radiosurgery alone, with WBRT reserved for salvage, has been proposed. However, even under ideal circumstances with focal treatments, microscopic disease may remain. The aim of adjuvant WBRT is to eradicate any residual disease to enhance local control, both at the focal site and in the rest of the brain. Defining the best approach in regard to the timing and sequence of these modalities remains has been the subject of two studies.

Resection Alone

There is only one randomized prospective trial examining the benefit of adjuvant WBRT following resection (Table 4) [14]. In this study, Patchell et al. randomized 95 patients with a single brain metastasis to resection with post-operative WBRT (n = 49) to a total dose of 50.4 Gy in 28 fractions or no post-operative WBRT (n = 46). Patients who received post-operative WBRT had significantly decreased overall intracranial failure (18 vs. 70%, p < 0.001) as well as decreased recurrence

Table 4. Prospective studies of focal treatment plus WBRT vs. focal treatment alone in patients with brain metastases

Study	Treatment	n	MOS	IF	Salvage Tx
Patchell et al. [14]	Surgery + WBRT vs.	49	48 weeks	18%	Not reported
	Surgery alone	46	43 weeks	70%	
			p = 0.39	p < 0.001	
Aoyama et al. [46]	Radiosurgery + WBRT vs.	67	7.5 months	46.8%	14.9%
	Radiosurgery alone	65	8.0 months	76.4%	44.6%
			p = 0.42	p < 0.001	p < 0.001

WBRT, whole brain radiation therapy; n, number of patients; MOS, median overall survival; IF, intracranial failure; Tx, treatment.

at the site of the original tumor bed (10 vs. 46%, $p < 0.001$) and elsewhere in the brain (14 vs. 37%, $p < 0.01$). This result underscores the superiority of adjuvant WBRT. Many detractors of WBRT however, quote that there was no difference between the 2 arms in regard to overall survival (48 vs. 43 weeks, $p = 0.39$). The trial, in fact, was never powered to detect a change in the survival endpoint and therefore using the survival endpoint from this trial to augment the argument to withhold WBRT is simply untenable. Further, salvage WBRT was given to 61% of patients in the surgery only arm, further clouding the results; additionally, the usage of salvage WBRT occurred very early, suggesting that no meaningful delay of WBRT usage was achieved. While half of those patients who received surgery alone and WBRT at relapse died of CNS recurrence, only 14% of patients treated with surgery followed by WBRT had CNS recurrence as a cause of death, implying that salvage WBRT is significantly inferior to upfront WBRT. It is important to note that patients who received both surgery and WBRT had a survival of 12 months, nearly 2–3 times greater than historical values [41]. Because of the inferior local control resulting from withholding WBRT after resection, adjuvant WBRT following resection is advised. This topic is discussed in more detail in Chapter 5, Surgery for Brain Metastases.

Radiosurgery Alone

The use of radiosurgery alone was first examined in a series of retrospective reports that demonstrated equivalent median survival in patients receiving radiosurgery alone compared to radiosurgery and WBRT [42–45]. However, in all of these series, patients receiving WBRT had improved local control, compared to radiosurgery alone. These studies were retrospective and treatment assignment was not randomized, resulting in patient selection bias.

The Japanese Radiotherapy Oncology Group recently published the results of a multi-institutional, prospective, randomized trial investigating this question in patients with 4 or fewer brain metastases (Table 4) [46]. In this study, 132 patients with lesions less than 3 cm were randomized to receive radiosurgery alone (n = 67) or radiosurgery followed by WBRT (n = 65). Local control was significantly enhanced in patients treated with WBRT with a 12-month intracranial recurrence rate of 46.8% in the WBRT plus radiosurgery arm vs. 76.4% in the radiosurgery alone arm (p < 0.001). Median survival was equivalent in both arms (7.5 vs. 8.0 months, p = 0.42), but once again, most statisticians would consider an n of 132 as being inadequate to truly assess a survival difference. Salvage treatment was less frequently used in patients who received WBRT compared to radiosurgery alone. Death due to a neurologic cause occurred in 22.8% of patients in the WBRT plus radiosurgery arm compared to 19.3% in the radiosurgery alone arm (p = 0.64). Differences in systemic and neurologic functional preservation and radiation toxicities were not found, underscoring the fact that WBRT did not result in measurably greater neurologic deterioration. Another co-operative inter-group trial is also investigating this strategy in a prospective randomized trial that aims to accrue 480 patients over a period of 5 years.

The results of these trials provide evidence favoring the use of adjuvant WBRT to improve local and intracranial control. A small phase II prospective study of the Eastern Cooperative Oncology Group investigated the use of radiosurgery alone in patients with tumors considered radioresistant, melanoma, renal cell carcinoma, and sarcoma [47]. Median survival was found to be 8.2 months in the 31 assessable patients. More importantly, significant rates of local and intracranial relapse were identified, suggesting that withholding WBRT maybe detrimental.

Utility of Adjuvant WBRT

A current practice concept contends that the comparable survival found in the trials described above is enough to justify reserving WBRT for salvage despite the improved intracranial control with immediate adjuvant WBRT. Table 4 reviews the results of these trials. Those in favor of this approach propose that patients with limited amount of disease (3–10 lesions, depending on the institution) be treated with focal treatment alone and be subsequently followed by serial imaging. If a new intracranial lesion appears, it is treated with focal treatment again (usually radiosurgery). Proponents of this approach cite the putative high rates of neurotoxicity associated with WBRT as additional rationale.

DeAngelis et al. published the results of a small trial demonstrating an 11% risk of developing dementia based on the retrospective review of 47 patients with brain metastases treated with WBRT [48]. These patients were considered long-term survivors (greater than 12 months). However these patients received doses higher than today's standard. Of the 15 patients included in this report treated with regimens used today, none developed dementia. Furthermore, it has been suggested more recently that decline in neurocognitive function and neurologic deficits were likely present before receiving WBRT and that WBRT alone does not result in significant neuropsychological decline [49]. The recent phase III trial by the Japanese Radiotherapy Oncology Group reported no difference neurologic function in patients treated with radiosurgery alone compared to those treated with radiosurgery followed by immediate adjuvant WBRT [46].

Preventing recurrent disease has also been found to be important in preserving neurocognitive status and may outweigh the potential toxicities of WBRT. Patients with recurrent brain metastases have been found to have decreased mental performance and increased neurological deficits [50, 51]. Additionally, progressive disease as detected by MRI has been shown to result in increased neurocognitive deterioration [52]. Neurocognitive impairment represents a key issue in radiotherapy for patients with brain metastases and is discussed further below.

In summary, the importance of superior local control as demonstrated in patients receiving adjuvant WBRT cannot be understated, especially in patients with controlled systemic disease. Impact of salvage therapy with WBRT cannot be ignored in these trials (Table 4). The risk of permanent adverse effects from WBRT must be weighed against the adverse effects that accompany tumor recurrence. Furthermore, serial imaging and re-treatment with radiosurgery dramatically increases the overall cost of managing these patients as imaging studies can cost at least $2,000 per study and radiosurgical procedures cost approximately $20,000 – 40,000. In the absence of evidence to substantiate claims that omission of WBRT results in decreased toxicity and improved quality of life, immediate adjuvant WBRT should remain the standard of care in patients receiving focal treatment. The suggestion of equivalent survival in these trials comes from lack of appropriate power to detect a survival difference and cannot be substantiated based on the small patient numbers.

Neurocognitive Function

With the relatively poor performance status and short overall survival found in the majority of patients with brain metastases, outcomes such as neurocognitive function and quality of life are important to consider. These measures will become increasingly significant with the advent of newer treatments prolonging survival. This belief was reflected in a current survey where a majority of medical and radiation oncologists (74%) responded that managing neurologic and neurocognitive function was more important than prolonging survival in patients with brain metastases [53].

Neurocognitive dysfunction may be caused by radiotherapy, systemic treatment such as chemotherapy and hormonal agents, surgery, adjuvant medications and the tumor itself. Neurocognitive deficits following radiotherapy are divided into acute, subacute, and late toxicities. Acute toxicities are caused by cerebral edema, resulting in drowsiness, headache, nausea, vomiting, and focal defects. They present within the first few weeks of treatment and are generally reversible. Appearing 1–6 months after treatment are subacute effects, which are thought to be the result of diffuse demyelination, manifesting as headache, somnolence, and fatigability. Late effects

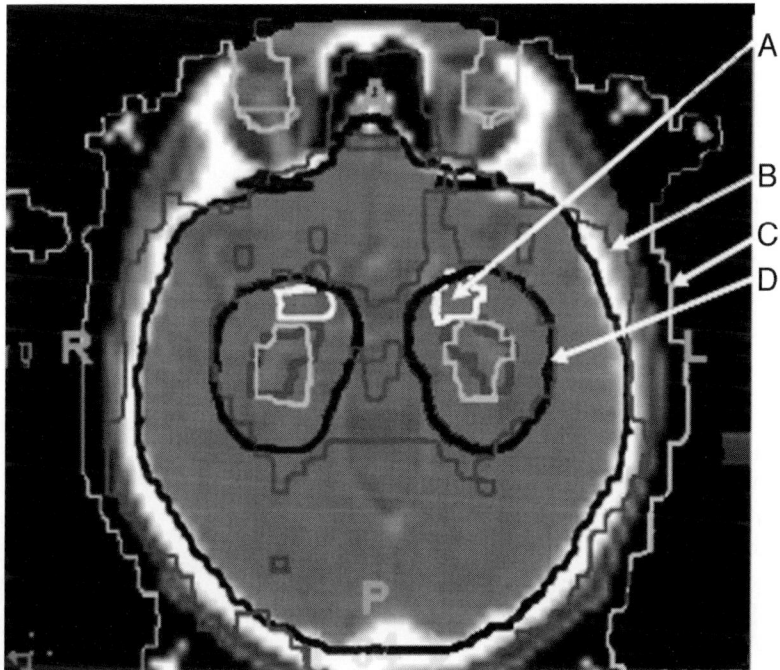

Figure 1. Hippocampus avoidance plan with intensity modulated radiotherapy via helical tomotherapy: A. Avoidance region (white); B. 30 Gy (dark grey) ; C. 6 Gy (light grey); D. 3 Gy (black).

appear after 6 months, secondary to vascular injury, demyelination, and necrosis. Clinically, patients may show mild lassitude, memory impairment, or dementia that may be irreversible and progressive.

While the precise incidence of neurocognitive deficits in patients with brain metastases is unknown due to differences in treatment regimens and patient characteristics from the few reporting centers, most studies report that cognitive dysfunction is present in the majority of patients before receiving radiotherapy [49, 54, 55]. A recent phase III trial of 401 patients reported baseline cognitive impairment in 91% of patients [56].

Neurocognitive function has recently been linked to survival, progression of disease, and radiographic response to WBRT. Baseline neurocognitive function has been demonstrated to be predictive of survival [56, 57]. Investigators observed that cognitive deterioration occurred around 6 weeks prior to radiographic failure, suggesting that neurocognitive function may be predictive of failure [52]. Additionally, patients responding to WBRT as volumetrically measured on MRI (66% reduction or greater) have been found to have better neurocognitive function and longer survival [58].

Approaches to improve neurocognitive function include pharmacologic agents and modifications to the delivery of WBRT. Methylphenidate, donepezil, and memantine have been used with modestly promising results [59–62]. Patients receiving doses of greater then 3 Gy per fraction have been shown to be at higher risk for developing dementia in the long-term, so hypofractionation regimens should be avoided[48]. A preclinical study in rats showed that doses as low as 2 Gy or less can damage the hippocampus, especially the neural stem cell population in the subventricular and the subgranular zones[63]. Avoidance of the hippocampus using conformal radiotherapy is currently being investigated as shown in Figure 1 [64]. This technology allows for full dose to the majority of the brain while limiting the dose to the hippocampus, potentially sparing the exquisitely radiosensitive neural stem cell population capable of generating migratory cells involved in repair and plasticity of brain function.

In summary, as some patients with brain metastases are surviving longer, understanding neurocognitive function has become increasingly important. Treatments with pharmacologic agents and modifications to radiotherapy are currently being examined in clinical trials. Further data are needed for validation of these approaches.

Brachytherapy

Brachytherapy, which delivers radiation locally in or near the tumor through the use of radioactive seed implants, radioactive colloids inserted into tumor-associated cysts, or inflatable balloon catheters placed in the lesion or surgical cavity, is another method of delivering radiation. An advantage of this approach is the ability to deliver higher doses directly to the targeted area while limiting exposure to the surrounding area. Treatment is generally well-tolerated and potential adverse effects include wound and bone flap infection, and cerebrospinal fluid leak, as well as late necrosis.

Data are limited examining the use of ^{125}I implants in patients with brain metastases [65–68]. While brachytherapy has been replaced by radiosurgery in general, it may still have a role in patients with larger (greater than 3 cm) lesions [69]. No prospective, randomized trials have been reported. A new method using an inflatable balloon catheter containing a temporary liquid ^{125}I radiation source has been studied in primary brain tumors and more recently in patients with brain metastases [70]. The use of brachytherapy in patients with brain metastases has yet to be fully defined.

Chemical Modifiers

Along with advances in the delivery of radiotherapy, the addition of systemic agents to radiotherapy is another strategy to enhance the effects of treatment. Recently developed radiosensitizers and chemotherapeutic agents have demonstrated promising results, especially in a subsets of patients. These compounds are thought to have a synergistic effect when used in conjunction with radiotherapy. The optimal combination, including timing and sequence, is currently being investigated.

Radiosensitizers

Radiosensitizers are designed to increase the efficacy of radiotherapy in malignant tissue without additional damage to normal tissue. Historically, radiosensitizers have demonstrated little value in patients with brain metastases. Misonidazole, bromodeoxyuridine (BUdR), and other agents have failed to show significant benefit in randomized trials [71, 72]. The development of 2 new compounds, motexafin gadolinium (MGd) and efaproxiril (RSR-13), have renewed interest in this strategy.

Motexafin Gadolinium

MGd is a redox modulator that works by generating reactive oxygen species. The increased reactive oxygen species deplete the stores of reducing agents needed for repair of cytotoxic damage, thereby enhancing radiotherapy-induced apoptosis [73]. This agent selectively concentrates in malignant tissue as shown by MRI (see Figure 2) [56, 74]. Early studies showed response rates of 68–72% in patients with brain metastases treated with MGd and WBRT [74, 75].

A phase III prospective randomized controlled trial compared WBRT alone (30 Gy in 10 fractions) to WBRT with MGd (5 mg/kg/day) in 401 patients [76].

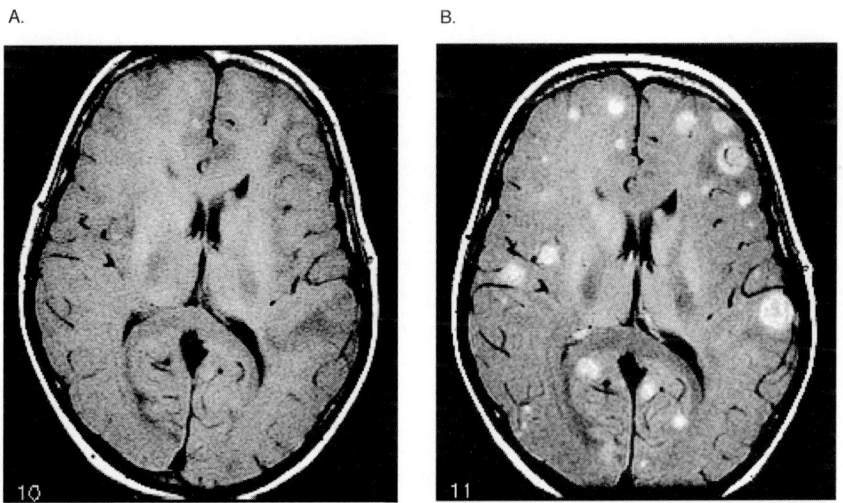

Figure 2. Magnetic resonance imaging of a patient with brain metastases: A. Noncontrast scan at baseline; B. Noncontrast scan after administration of motexafin gadolinium.

Patients were stratified according to primary tumor histology, RPA class, and study center. There was no significant difference in the primary endpoints of median survival (5.2 vs. 4.9 months, p = 0.48) and median time to neurologic progression (9.5 vs. 8.3 months, p = 0.95). However, when tumor type was examined, an increased time to neurologic progression was found in the 63% of patients with non-small cell lung cancer treated with MGd compared to those who received WBRT alone (median not reached vs. 7.4 months, p = 0.048). A significant improvement in the secondary endpoints of death from CNS causes and memory and executive function was also demonstrated in the MGd arm for patients with non-small cell lung cancer. Adverse events were mild to moderate and easily manageable and administration of MGd did not interfere with delivery of radiotherapy.

A confirmatory phase III trial investigating the use of MGd in patients with brain metastases and NSCLC primaries has been completed and results were recently presented at the American Society of Therapeutic Radiation Oncology [77]. In this international multi-center prospective trial, 554 patients were randomized to receive WBRT alone (n = 275) or WBRT with MGd (n = 279). There was a trend toward an improvement in the primary endpoint, time to neurologic progression, in patients who received WBRT plus MGd compared to WBRT alone that was not found to be significant (15.4 vs. 10 months, p = 0.12). On further analysis of patients by region, patients treated in North America, a significant prolongation of both time to neurologic and neurocognitive progression was observed in patients treated with WBRT and MGd. Patients treated in North America received WBRT sooner after diagnosis of brain metastases then patients in Europe and Australia (median 1.6 weeks vs. 3.1 weeks) as patients outside of North America were more often treated initially with chemotherapy. A significant improvement in time to neurologic progression was found in patients who received WBRT within 3 weeks of diagnosis of brain metastases regardless of region, in patients whose lung cancer as newly diagnosed, in patients who never received chemotherapy prior to randomization, and in patients in RTOG RPA class II.

In addition to these direct therapeutic benefits, MGd may be useful as a diagnostic tool. MGd has been recently shown to identify occult lesions previously undetected using standard gadolinium contrast agents on MRI in 1/3 of patients in a recent phase II trial [78]. These results suggest that a proportion of patients with their treatment designed using standard imaging may be undertreated. While MGd has shown promising results in a subset of patients, its precise role in the diagnosis and treatment of brain metastases remains undefined.

Efaproxaril

Efaproxiril, an allosteric modifier, binds non-covalently to hemoglobin and decreases its oxygen binding affinity thereby increasing tissue pO2. Efaproxaril with WBRT was examined in 57 patients with brain metastases who received WBRT (30 Gy in 10 fractions) and efaproxaril (100 mg/kg) along with supplemental oxygen at 4 liters given before, during, and after delivery of a fraction [79]. These patients were compared retrospectively to a matched cohort from the RTOG RPA brain metastases database. Median survival was found to be significantly improved for the efaproxaril-treated patients (6.4 vs. 4.1 months, p = 0.0174). A prospective randomized trial did not confirm this survival benefit. In this phase III study, in 538 patients with brain metastases in RPA class 1 or 2 were randomized to WBRT (30 Gy in 10 fractions) or WBRT with efaproxaril [80]. No significant difference in the primary endpoint of survival was shown (5.3 vs. 4.5 months, p = 0.17). Interestingly, on further analysis of tumor type, patients with breast cancer (21%) demonstrated improved survival when treated with efaproxaril compared to WBRT alone (8.7 vs. 4.6 months, p = 0.061). Further investigation of this observation is underway with the ENRICH trial which recently completed enrolling women with breast cancer. Routine use of this agent cannot be recommended at this time in the absence of further clinical data.

Chemotherapy

Combining chemotherapy with radiotherapy represents another multimodal approach in the treatment of brain metastases. The timing of combination chemotherapy with WBRT varies with region with the majority of patients in North America receiving WBRT soon after diagnosis. Patients in Europe, especially France, often receive upfront chemotherapy [77]. This question has been evaluated in a small phase III study by Robinet et al. [81]. One hundred seventy-six patients with brain metastases from non-small cell lung cancer were randomized to receive chemotherapy with cisplatin and vinorelbine followed by delayed or early WBRT. They found no significant difference in survival between the 2 arms (24 vs. 21 weeks, p = 0.83), which is not surprising due to the high rate of death due to extracranial progression in these patients. However, response rates of brain metastases in these trials are similar to the expected response rates for the primary tumor [82, 83].

This section will highlight chemotherapeutic agents that have been investigated for use in conjunction with radiotherapy such as temozolomide and interstitial 1,3-Bis(2-Chloroethyl)-1-Nitrosourea (BCNU). Further discussion on chemotherapy can be found in Chapters 10 and 11, Chemotherapy for Brain Metastases: Solid Tumors: Lung Cancer, GI Malignancies, Melanoma/Dermatologic Malignancies; and Chemotherapy for Brain Metastases: Solid Tumors: Breast Cancer, GYN Malignancies, Musculoskeletal Tumors, respectively.

Temozolomide

Temozolomide is a newly developed oral alkylating agent that has shown significant survival benefit when given concomitantly and adjuvantly with radiotherapy in patients with Grade IV gliomas with minimally toxicity [84]. It is able to effectively penetrate the blood-brain barrier because of its small molecular size and lipophilic properties. It can achieve cerebrospinal concentrations of approximately 30% of plasma concentrations with almost 100% bioavailability [85]. When used alone, it has shown modest activity in recurrent and newly diagnosed brain metastases [86–91]. In preclinical studies, temozolomide has been found to have a synergistic effect with radiation [92].

Concomitant chemoradiotherapy with temozolomide in patients with brain metastases has been investigated in phase II and III trials [93–95]. In a phase II trial by Antonadou et al., patients randomized to receive WBRT (40 Gy in 20 fractions) plus concomitant (75 mg/m2/day) and adjuvant (200 mg/m2/day on days 1–5 every 38 days) temozolomide demonstrated a significantly higher response rate than patients receiving WBRT alone (96% [38% CR, 58% PR] vs. 66% [33% CR, 33% PR] p = 0.017) [93]. Treatment was well-tolerated. Another phase II study by Verger observed contradictory results with no significant difference in radiographic response in patients treated with WBRT alone or WBRT combined with concurrent and adjuvant temozolomide [94]. However, progression free survival at 90 days was superior in the temozolomide group compared to the WBRT alone group (72 vs. 54%, p = 0.03). Rate of neurologic death was improved in the temozolomide arm as well (41 vs. 69%, p = 0.029). The largest study is a phase III trial by Antonadou et al. that randomized 134 patients to WBRT alone (30 Gy in 10 fractions) or WBRT with concomitant and adjuvant temozolomide at the doses described above [95]. Response rate was significantly improved in the temozolomide arm (53 vs. 33%, p = 0.039). The benefit was more pronounced in patients less than 60 years old (77 vs. 32%, p = 0.003) and those with a Karnofsky performance status of 90 or greater (71 vs. 32%, p = 0.003). There was no significant difference in survival (8.3 vs. 6.3 months, p = 0.179). These trials suggest a benefit with the addition of concomitant and adjuvant temozolomide to WBRT, but further data are needed to warrant treatment with temozolomide as standard practice.

Interstitial Chemotherapy

Interstitial chemotherapy allows the introduction of chemotherapeutic agents directly into the resection cavity following surgery. A biodegradable polymer containing BCNU (Gliadel wafer) is the only interstitial chemotherapy treatment approved currently for recurrent and newly diagnosed malignant gliomas. This treatment combined with surgery and WBRT has been evaluated in an early clinical trial [96]. This series included 42 patients with brain metastases, 81% newly diagnosed and 75% with lung and melanoma primary histologies, who were treated with maximal surgical resection followed by implantable BCNU wafers, and WBRT to 30 to 44 Gy. Local control was 100% in newly patients with newly diagnosed lesions with a mean survival of 16.8 months. Nine patients (22%) were still alive with no evidence of recurrent central nervous system disease. Larger, prospective, randomized trials are needed to further define the role of this treatment.

Recommendations and Conclusion

Despite advances in treatment delivery, median survival has remained fixed at 4 to 6 months. Definitive WBRT remains the standard of care for the majority of patients, especially those with multiple lesions. The application of multi-modal approaches such as resection, radiosurgery, and chemical modifiers with WBRT has been investigated with promising results.

For patients with a single metastasis, resection or radiosurgery combined with WBRT has been shown to increase survival in large phase III trials, thus providing level 1 evidence to justify these approaches as the new standard of care in these patients. Since there has never been a prospective randomized trial directly comparing resection and radiosurgery, a definitive recommendation cannot be made regarding the indications for each modality. Radiosurgery is useful in patients who have a lesion that impinges on an eloquent area or those who are unable to tolerate surgery. Surgical resection may be preferred when the diagnosis is in doubt, when immediate relief of major increase in intracranial pressure is necessary, and when the lesion is large (greater than 3–4 cm). These recommendations are supported by the results of 2 recent meta-analyses [97, 98].

Although focal treatment such as resection and radiosurgery with WBRT have purportedly shown equivalent survival compared to focal treatment alone in phase III trials, local control is definitely improved with the addition of WBRT, and the trials were too small to genuinely answer the survival question. Control of intracranial disease is especially important in patients with controlled extracranial disease. Furthermore, the risk of permanent adverse effects from recurrent disease must be balanced with the toxicities that accompany WBRT, most of which are reversible or uncommon. Until evidence is produced substantiating the claim the omission of WBRT results in an improved clinical outcome, immediate adjuvant WBRT should remain standard of care in patients receiving local treatment.

Future trials in patients should consider quality of life measures such as neurocognitive function. While neurocognitive dysfunction is present before treatment in the majority of patients, resection, radiotherapy, and systemic agents may worsen symptoms. Strategies to improve neurocognitive function such as pharmacologic therapies and radiotherapy modifications are under investigation.

Chemical modifiers represent another area of great interest in the multi-modal approach to patients with brain metastases. MGd has shown to improve outcomes in a subset of patients. Temozolomide with WBRT has shown promise in early clinical trials and may act synergistically with radiation. Further data are awaited before routine administration of these agents is recommended.

While our understanding of brain metastases and radiotherapy has improved substantially over the past 30 years, a dramatic improvement in outcome has not been demonstrated. Large, well-designed, prospective, randomized trials that consider other endpoints in addition to survival such as neurologic and neurocognitive function are needed to further define treatment. Until then, the trials described above should guide treatment.

References

1. Andrews DW, Scott CB, Sperduto PW, et al. Whole brain radiation therapy with or without stereotactic radiosurgery boost for patients with one to three brain metastases: phase III results of the RTOG 9508 randomised trial. Lancet 2004;363:1665–72.

2. Patchell RA, Tibbs PA, Walsh JW, et al. A randomized trial of surgery in the treatment of single metastases to the brain. N Engl J Med 1990;322:494–500.

3. Noordijk EM, Vecht CJ, Haaxma-Reiche H, et al. The choice of treatment of single brain metastasis should be based on extracranial tumor activity and age. Int J Radiat Oncol Biol Phys 1994;29:711–7.

4. Chao JH, Phillips R, Nickson JJ. Roentgen-ray therapy of cerebral metastases. Cancer 1954;7:682–9.

5. Lang EF, Slater J. Metastatic Brain Tumors. Results of Surgical and Nonsurgical Treatment. Surg Clin North Am 1964;44:865–72.

6. Richards P, Mc KW. Intracranial metastases. Br Med J 1963;5322:15–8.

7. Borgelt B, Gelber R, Kramer S, et al. The palliation of brain metastases: final results of the first two studies by the Radiation Therapy Oncology Group. Int J Radiat Oncol Biol Phys 1980;6:1–9.

8. Gaspar L, Scott C, Rotman M, et al. Recursive partitioning analysis (RPA) of prognostic factors in three Radiation Therapy Oncology Group (RTOG) brain metastases trials. Int J Radiat Oncol Biol Phys 1997;37:745–51.

9. Sze G, Mehta M, Schultz CJ. Radiologic response evaluation of brain metastases: uni-dimensional World Health Organization (WHO) response evaluation criteria in solid tumors (RECIST) vs dimensional or 3-dimensional criteria. Proc Am Soc Clin Oncol 2001;20:59a.

10. Nieder C, Berberich W, Schnabel K. Tumor-related prognostic factors for remission of brain metastases after radiotherapy. Int J Radiat Oncol Biol Phys 1997;39:25–30.

11. Mahmoud-Ahmed AS, Kupelian PA, Reddy CA, et al. Brain metastases from gynecological cancers: factors that affect overall survival. Technol Cancer Res Treat 2002;1:305–10.

12. Buchsbaum JC, Suh JH, Lee SY, et al. Survival by radiation therapy oncology group recursive partitioning analysis class and treatment modality in patients with brain metastases from malignant melanoma: a retrospective study. Cancer 2002;94:2265–72.

13. Arbit E, Wronski M, Burt M, et al. The treatment of patients with recurrent brain metastases. A retrospective analysis of 109 patients with nonsmall cell lung cancer. Cancer 1995;76:765–73.

14. Patchell RA, Tibbs PA, Regine WF, et al. Postoperative radiotherapy in the treatment of single metastases to the brain: a randomized trial. Jama 1998;280:1485–9.

15. Kondziolka D, Patel A, Lunsford LD, et al. Stereotactic radiosurgery plus whole brain radiotherapy versus radiotherapy alone for patients with multiple brain metastases. Int J Radiat Oncol Biol Phys 1999;45:427–34.
16. Gaspar LE, Scott C, Murray K, et al. Validation of the RTOG recursive partitioning analysis (RPA) classification for brain metastases. Int J Radiat Oncol Biol Phys 2000;47:1001–6.
17. Harwood AR, Simson WJ. Radiation therapy of cerebral metastases: a randomized prospective clinical trial. Int J Radiat Oncol Biol Phys 1977;2:1091–4.
18. Kurtz JM, Gelber R, Brady LW, et al. The palliation of brain metastases in a favorable patient population: a randomized clinical trial by the Radiation Therapy Oncology Group. Int J Radiat Oncol Biol Phys 1981;7:891–5.
19. Borgelt B, Gelber R, Larson M, et al. Ultra-rapid high dose irradiation schedules for the palliation of brain metastases: final results of the first two studies by the Radiation Therapy Oncology Group. Int J Radiat Oncol Biol Phys 1981;7:1633–8.
20. Chatani M, Teshima T, Hata K, et al. Prognostic factors in patients with brain metastases from lung carcinoma. Strahlenther Onkol 1986;162:157–61.
21. Haie-Meder C, Pellae-Cosset B, Laplanche A, et al. Results of a randomized clinical trial comparing two radiation schedules in the palliative treatment of brain metastases. Radiother Oncol 1993;26:111–6.
22. Chatani M, Matayoshi Y, Masaki N, et al. Radiation therapy for brain metastases from lung carcinoma. Prospective randomized trial according to the level of lactate dehydrogenase. Strahlenther Onkol 1994;170:155–61.
23. Murray KJ, Scott C, Greenberg HM, et al. A randomized phase III study of accelerated hyperfractionation versus standard in patients with unresected brain metastases: a report of the Radiation Therapy Oncology Group (RTOG) 9104. Int J Radiat Oncol Biol Phys 1997;39:571–4.
24. Epstein BE, Scott CB, Sause WT, et al. Improved survival duration in patients with unresected solitary brain metastasis using accelerated hyperfractionated radiation therapy at total doses of 54.4 gray and greater. Results of Radiation Therapy Oncology Group 85–28. Cancer 1993;71:1362–7.
25. Sause WT, Scott C, Krisch R, et al. Phase I/II trial of accelerated fractionation in brain metastases RTOG 85–28. Int J Radiat Oncol Biol Phys 1993;26: 653–7.
26. Bezjak A, Adam J, Barton R, et al. Symptom response after palliative radiotherapy for patients with brain metastases. Eur J Cancer 2002;38:487–96.
27. Mintz AH, Kestle J, Rathbone MP, et al. A randomized trial to assess the efficacy of surgery in addition to radiotherapy in patients with a single cerebral metastasis. Cancer 1996;78:1470–6.
28. Bindal RK, Sawaya R, Leavens ME, et al. Surgical treatment of multiple brain metastases. J Neurosurg 1993;79:210–6.
29. Auchter RM, Lamond JP, Alexander E, et al. A multiinstitutional outcome and prognostic factor analysis of radiosurgery for resectable single brain metastasis. Int J Radiat Oncol Biol Phys 1996;35:27–35.

30. Shaw E, Scott C, Souhami L, et al. Single dose radiosurgical treatment of recurrent previously irradiated primary brain tumors and brain metastases: final report of RTOG protocol 90–05. Int J Radiat Oncol Biol Phys 2000;47:291–8.
31. Petrovich Z, Yu C, Giannotta SL, et al. Survival and pattern of failure in brain metastasis treated with stereotactic gamma knife radiosurgery. J Neurosurg 2002;97:499–506.
32. Mehta MP, Patel RR. Radiotherapy & radiosurger for brain metastases. In: Black PM, Loeffler JS, eds. Cancer of the Central Nervous System. 2nd ed. Philadelphia: Lippincott Williams & Wilkins; 2001.
33. Flickinger JC, Kondziolka D, Lunsford LD, et al. A multi-institutional experience with stereotactic radiosurgery for solitary brain metastasis. Int J Radiat Oncol Biol Phys 1994;28:797–802.
34. Alexander E, 3rd, Moriarty TM, Davis RB, et al. Stereotactic radiosurgery for the definitive, noninvasive treatment of brain metastases. J Natl Cancer Inst 1995;87:34–40.
35. Chougule PB, Burton-Williams M, Saris S, et al. Randomized treatment of brain metastasis with gamma knife radiosurgery, whole brain radiotherapy, or both. Int J Radiat Oncol Biol Phys 2000;48:114.
36. Sanghavi SN, Miranpuri SS, Chappell R, et al. Radiosurgery for patients with brain metastases: a multi-institutional analysis, stratified by the RTOG recursive partitioning analysis method. Int J Radiat Oncol Biol Phys 2001;51:426–34.
37. Bhatnagar AK, Flickinger JC, Kondziolka D, et al. Stereotactic radiosurgery for four or more intracranial metastases. Int J Radiat Oncol Biol Phys 2006; 64:898–903.
38. Bindal AK, Bindal RK, Hess KR, et al. Surgery versus radiosurgery in the treatment of brain metastasis. J Neurosurg 1996;84:748–54.
39. O'Neill BP, Iturria NJ, Link MJ, et al. A comparison of surgical resection and stereotactic radiosurgery in the treatment of solitary brain metastases. Int J Radiat Oncol Biol Phys 2003;55:1169–76.
40. Mehta M, Noyes W, Craig B, et al. A cost-effectiveness and cost-utility analysis of radiosurgery vs. resection for single-brain metastases. Int J Radiat Oncol Biol Phys 1997;39:445–54.
41. Patchell RA, Regine WF. The rationale for adjuvant whole brain radiation therapy with radiosurgery in the treatment of single brain metastases. Technol Cancer Res Treat 2003;2:111–5.
42. Sneed PK, Suh JH, Goetsch SJ, et al. A multi-institutional review of radiosurgery alone vs. radiosurgery with whole brain radiotherapy as the initial management of brain metastases. International Journal of Radiation Oncology, Biology, Physics 2002;53:519–26.
43. Sneed PK, Lamborn KR, Forstner JM, et al. Radiosurgery for brain metastases: is whole brain radiotherapy necessary? International Journal of Radiation Oncology, Biology, Physics 1999;43:549–58.

44. Hoffman R, Sneed PK, McDermott MW, et al. Radiosurgery for brain metastases from primary lung carcinoma. Cancer J 2001;7:121–31.
45. Pirzkall A, Debus J, Lohr F, et al. Radiosurgery alone or in combination with whole-brain radiotherapy for brain metastases. Journal of Clinical Oncology 1998;16:3563–9.
46. Aoyama H, Shirato H, Tago M, et al. Stereotactic radiosurgery plus whole-brain radiation therapy vs stereotactic radiosurgery alone for treatment of brain metastases: a randomized controlled trial. Jama 2006;295:2483–91.
47. Manon RR, O'Neill A, Mehta MP, et al. Phase II trial of radiosurgery (RS) for 1 to 3 newly diagnosed brain metastases from renal cell, melanoma, and sarcoma (An Eastern Cooperative Oncology Group Study (E6397)). Proc Am Soc Clin Incol 2004;22:108S.
48. DeAngelis LM, Delattre JY, Posner JB. Radiation-induced dementia in patients cured of brain metastases. Neurology 1989;39:789–96.
49. Penitzka S, Steinvorth S, Sehlleier S, et al. [Assessment of cognitive function after preventive and therapeutic whole brain irradiation using neuropsychological testing]. Strahlenther Onkol 2002;178:252–8.
50. Regine WF, Scott C, Murray K, et al. Neurocognitive outcome in brain metastases patients treated with accelerated-fractionation vs. accelerated-hyperfractionated radiotherapy: an analysis from Radiation Therapy Oncology Group Study 91–04. Int J Radiat Oncol Biol Phys 2001;51:711–7.
51. Regine WF, Huhn JL, Patchell RA, et al. Risk of symptomatic brain tumor recurrence and neurologic deficit after radiosurgery alone in patients with newly diagnosed brain metastases: results and implications. Int J Radiat Oncol Biol Phys 2002;52:333–8.
52. Meyers CA, Hess KR. Multifaceted end points in brain tumor clinical trials: cognitive deterioration precedes MRI progression. Neuro-oncol 2003; 5:89–95.
53. Renschler MF, Mehta MP, Donald DM, et al. Treatment intent for brain metastases: Surveys of medical and radiation oncologists indicate that maintaining neurologic and neurocognitive function is more important that prolonging survival. Proc Am Soc Clin Oncol 2003;22:552.
54. Gregor A, Cull A, Stephens RJ, et al. Prophylactic cranial irradiation is indicated following complete response to induction therapy in small cell lung cancer: results of a multicentre randomised trial. United Kingdom Coordinating Committee for Cancer Research (UKCCCR) and the European Organization for Research and Treatment of Cancer (EORTC). Eur J Cancer 1997;33:1752–8.
55. Komaki R, Meyers CA, Shin DM, et al. Evaluation of cognitive function in patients with limited small cell lung cancer prior to and shortly following prophylactic cranial irradiation. Int J Radiat Oncol Biol Phys 1995;33:179–82.
56. Meyers CA, Smith JA, Bezjak A, et al. Neurocognitive function and progression in patients with brain metastases treated with whole-brain radiation and motexafin gadolinium: results of a randomized phase III trial. J Clin Oncol 2004;22:157–65.

57. Meyers CA, Hess KR, Yung WK, et al. Cognitive function as a predictor of survival in patients with recurrent malignant glioma. J Clin Oncol 2000;18: 646–50.
58. Li J, Bentzen SM, Renschler M, et al. MRI response after whole brain radiation therapy in patients with brain metastases and its association with change in neurocognitive function. Int J Radiat Oncol Biol Phys 2006;66:S87.
59. Meyers CA, Weitzner MA, Valentine AD, et al. Methylphenidate therapy improves cognition, mood, and function of brain tumor patients. J Clin Oncol 1998;16:2522–7.
60. Rapp SR, Rosdhal R, D'Agostino RB, et al. Improving cognitive functioning in brain irradiated patients: a phase II trial of an acetylcholinesterase inhibitor (donepezil). Neuro-oncol 2004;6:357.
61. Pellegrini JW, Lipton SA. Delayed administration of memantine prevents N-methyl-D-aspartate receptor-mediated neurotoxicity. Ann Neurol 1993; 33:403–7.
62. Chen HS, Pellegrini JW, Aggarwal SK, et al. Open-channel block of N-methyl-D-aspartate (NMDA) responses by memantine: therapeutic advantage against NMDA receptor-mediated neurotoxicity. J Neurosci 1992;12:4427–36.
63. Peissner W, Kocher M, Treuer H, et al. Ionizing radiation-induced apoptosis of proliferating stem cells in the dentate gyrus of the adult rat hippocampus. Brain Res Mol Brain Res 1999;71:61–8.
64. Jaradat H, Khuntia D, Johnson S, et al. Whole-brain radiation treatment with hippocampal avoidance with tomotherapy. Neuro-oncol 2006;8:487.
65. Ostertag CB, Kreth FW. Interstitial iodine-125 radiosurgery for cerebral metastases. Br J Neurosurg 1995;9:593–603.
66. Bernstein M, Cabantog A, Laperriere N, et al. Brachytherapy for recurrent single brain metastasis. Can J Neurol Sci 1995;22:13–6.
67. Prados M, Leibel S, Barnett CM, et al. Interstitial brachytherapy for metastatic brain tumors. Cancer 1989;63:657–60.
68. Sneed PK, Stauffer PR, Gutin PH, et al. Interstitial irradiation and hyperthermia for the treatment of recurrent malignant brain tumors. Neurosurgery 1991;28:206–15.
69. Schulder M, Black PM, Shrieve DC, et al. Permanent low-activity iodine-125 implants for cerebral metastases. J Neurooncol 1997;33:213–21.
70. Tatter SB, Shaw EG, Rosenblum ML, et al. An inflatable balloon catheter and liquid 125I radiation source (GliaSite Radiation Therapy System) for treatment of recurrent malignant glioma: multicenter safety and feasibility trial. J Neurosurg 2003;99:297–303.
71. Komarnicky LT, Phillips TL, Martz K, et al. A randomized phase III protocol for the evaluation of misonidazole combined with radiation in the treatment of patients with brain metastases (RTOG-7916). Int J Radiat Oncol Biol Phys 1991;20:53–8.

72. Phillips TL, Scott CB, Leibel SA, et al. Results of a randomized comparison of radiotherapy and bromodeoxyuridine with radiotherapy alone for brain metastases: report of RTOG trial 89–05. Int J Radiat Oncol Biol Phys 1995;33: 339–48.

73. Khuntia D, Mehta M. Motexafin gadolinium: a clinical review of a novel radioenhancer for brain tumors. Expert Rev Anticancer Ther 2004;4:981–9.

74. Carde P, Timmerman R, Mehta MP, et al. Multicenter phase Ib/II trial of the radiation enhancer motexafin gadolinium in patients with brain metastases. J Clin Oncol 2001;19:2074–83.

75. Mehta MP, Shapiro WR, Glantz MJ, et al. Lead-in phase to randomized trial of motexafin gadolinium and whole-brain radiation for patients with brain metastases: centralized assessment of magnetic resonance imaging, neurocognitive, and neurologic end points. J Clin Oncol 2002;20:3445–53.

76. Mehta MP, Rodrigus P, Terhaard CH, et al. Survival and neurologic outcomes in a randomized trial of motexafin gadolinium and whole-brain radiation therapy in brain metastases. J Clin Oncol 2003;21:2529–36.

77. Mehta MP, Carrie C, Mahe MA, et al. Motexafin gadolinium (MGd) combined with prompt whole brain radiation therapy prolongs time to neurologic progressin in non-small cell lung cancer (NSCLC) patients with brain metastases: results of a randomized phase 3 trial. Int J Radiat Oncol Biol Phys 2006;66:S23.

78. Suh J, Mehta MP, Dagnault A, et al. Motexafin gadolinium-based treatment planning MRI identifies occult brain metastases amenable to stereotactic radiosurgery: Imaging results of a phase II trial of motexafin gadolinium and whole brain radiotherapy with stereotactic radiosurgery. Int J Radiat Oncol Biol Phys 2006;66:S193–4.

79. Shaw E, Scott C, Suh J, et al. RSR13 plus cranial radiation therapy in patients with brain metastases: comparison with the Radiation Therapy Oncology Group Recursive Partitioning Analysis Brain Metastases Database. J Clin Oncol 2003;21:2364–71.

80. Suh J, Stea B, Nabid A, et al. Standard whole brain radiation therapy (WBRT) with supplemental oxygen (O2), with or without RSR13 (efaproxiral)in patients with brain metastases: Results of the randomized REACH (RT-009) study. Proc Am Soc Clin Incol 2004;22:115S.

81. Robinet G, Thomas P, Breton JL, et al. Results of a phase III study of early versus delayed whole brain radiotherapy with concurrent cisplatin and vinorelbine combination in inoperable brain metastasis of non-small-cell lung cancer: Groupe Francais de Pneumo-Cancerologie (GFPC) Protocol 95–1. Ann Oncol 2001;12:59–67.

82. Bernardo G, Cuzzoni Q, Strada MR, et al. First-line chemotherapy with vinorelbine, gemcitabine, and carboplatin in the treatment of brain metastases from non-small-cell lung cancer: a phase II study. Cancer Invest 2002;20: 293–302.

83. Franciosi V, Cocconi G, Michiara M, et al. Front-line chemotherapy with cisplatin and etoposide for patients with brain metastases from breast carcinoma, nonsmall cell lung carcinoma, or malignant melanoma: a prospective study. Cancer 1999;85:1599–605.

84. Stupp R, Mason WP, van den Bent MJ, et al. Radiotherapy plus concomitant and adjuvant temozolomide for glioblastoma. N Engl J Med 2005;352:987–96.

85. Patel M, McCully C, Godwin K, et al. Plasma and cerebrospinal fluid pharmacokinetics of intravenous temozolomide in non-human primates. J Neurooncol 2003;61:203–7.

86. Abrey LE, Olson JD, Raizer JJ, et al. A phase II trial of temozolomide for patients with recurrent or progressive brain metastases. J Neurooncol 2001;53: 259–65.

87. Christodoulou C, Bafaloukos D, Kosmidis P, et al. Phase II study of temozolomide in heavily pretreated cancer patients with brain metastases. Ann Oncol 2001;12: 249–54.

88. Agarwala SS, Kirkwood JM, Gore M, et al. Temozolomide for the treatment of brain metastases associated with metastatic melanoma: a phase II study. J Clin Oncol 2004;22:2101–7.

89. Friedman HS, Evans B, Reardon D, et al. Phase II trial of temozolomide for patients with progressive brain metastases. Proc Am Soc Clin Oncol 2003; 22:102.

90. Dziadziuszko R, Ardizzoni A, Postmus PE, et al. Temozolomide in patients with advanced non-small cell lung cancer with and without brain metastases. a phase II study of the EORTC Lung Cancer Group (08965). Eur J Cancer 2003;39:1271–6.

91. Siena S, Landonia G, Baietta E, et al. Multicenter phase II study of temozolomide therapy for brain metastases in patients with malignant melanoma, breast cancer, and non-small cell lung cancer. Proc Am Soc Clin Oncol 2003;22:102.

92. Wedge SR, Porteous JK, Glaser MG, et al. In vitro evaluation of temozolomide combined with X-irradiation. Anticancer Drugs 1997;8:92–7.

93. Antonadou D, Paraskevaidis M, Sarris G, et al. Phase II randomized trial of temozolomide and concurrent radiotherapy in patients with brain metastases. J Clin Oncol 2002;20:3644–50.

94. Verger E, Gil M, Yaya R, et al. Temozolomide and concomitant whole brain radiotherapy in patients with brain metastases: a phase II randomized trial. Int J Radiat Oncol Biol Phys 2005;61:185–91.

95. Antonadou D, Coliarakis N, Paraskevaidis M, et al. Whole brain radiotherapy alone or in combination with temozolomide for brain metastases. A phase III study. Int J Radiat Oncol Biol Phys 2002;54:93.

96. Brem S, Staller A, Wotoczek-Obadia M. Interstitial chemotherapy for local control of CNS metastases. Neuro-oncol 2004;6:370–1.

97. Tsao MN, Lloyd NS, Wong RK, et al. Radiotherapeutic management of brain metastases: a systematic review and meta-analysis. Cancer Treat Rev 2005;31:256–73.
98. Stafinski T, Jhangri GS, Yan E, et al. Effectiveness of stereotactic radiosurgery alone or in combination with whole brain radiotherapy compared to conventional surgery and/or whole brain radiotherapy for the treatment of one or more brain metastases: a systematic review and meta-analysis. Cancer Treat Rev 2006;32:203–13.

7. Dural and Skull Base Metastases

Arnaldo Neves Da Silva, M.D. and David Schiff, M.D.

Dural Metastases

Introduction

Dural metastases (DM) usually affect patients in late stages of their disease with the majority of them harboring widespread metastatic disease that frequently accounts for the severity of the prognosis. They are also named pachymeningeal metastases and may arise from direct extension from skull metastasis or hematogenous spread from distant sites.

The incidence of DM has been progressively increasing over the past several decades as a result of the development of neuroimaging tools and prolonged patient survival as an effect of better cancer therapies [1].

DM are often asymptomatic but they can account for progressive neurological deficits. Occasionally the MRI can be misleading when the DM simulates a meningeal tumor or a subdural fluid collection masks the underlying tumor [2].

Epidemiology

Meyer and Reah in 1953 reviewing a necropsy series of 216 cases of central nervous system metastasis found 9.2% of patients had primary dural involvement [3]. Twenty per cent of their cases with diffuse dural metastases had concomitant leptomeningeal carcinomatosis and nearly half of the patients had associated subdural hemorrhages. Lung, breast, gastric and prostate cancers were equally common, with fewer cases of adrenal, unspecified bone and larynx cancers found.

In 1954, Lesse and Netsky found primary involvement of the meninges in 14.5% of 595 necropsies in patients who died of cancer [4]. In 40.6% of these patients the primary tumor was breast, with lung cancer in 9.3%. Prostate, multiple myeloma, malignant lymphomas, and leukemia were also observed.

The most referenced article is that of Posner and Chernik [5], who reviewed 2375 autopsies in patients with systemic cancer between 1970 and 1976. They identified

DM in 9% of the cases, the same percentage found by Meyer and Reah. They found DM from breast, prostate, neuroblastoma, Hodgkin's disease, non-Hodgkin's lymphoma, lung, and melanoma in decreasing order of frequency. Leptomeningeal carcinomatosis was found as commonly as DM. In 4% of DM patients the dural involvement was the only intracranial tumor site.

In contrast to the above series, Kleinschmidt-DeMasters did not find an overwhelming predominance of breast cancer metastasis in their series of surgical and autopsy cases [6–8]. This may reflect the improvements in treatment and survival time or tendency to forgo autopsy examination in patients with breast cancer in recent years.

Recently Laigle-Donadey [2] in an elegant literature review identified 198 published cases of dural metastasis between 1904 and 2003. The age of the patients ranged between 4 months and 84 years (mean age was 59 years). In decreasing order of frequency, prostate, breast, lung and stomach carcinomas encompassed 54.5% (108 patients), other carcinomas and hematological malignancies were also observed (table 1) [9–16]. The exact incidence of DM is difficult to evaluate because of the frequent combination with leptomeningeal disease.

Pathophysiology

Four mechanisms have been proposed to explain dural seeding: direct extension from calvarial metastasis, hematogenous dissemination, retrograde seeding through

Table 1. Cancer Types Disseminated to the Dura*

Cancer	Incidence (%)
Prostate	19.5
Breast	16.5
Lung	11
Gastric	7.5
Unknown	9.5
Hematologic	6.3

Incidence <5%

Renal	Seminoma
Colon/Rectal	Cervix/Endometrium
Neuroblastoma	Ewing's sarcoma
Pancreas	Other sarcomas
Hepatobiliary	Thymic
Carcinoid	Thyroid
Gallbladder	Choriocarcinoma
Urinary/bladder	Mesothelioma
Myeloma	

*Adapted from [2]

the valveless vertebral venous system (Batson's plexus), and least likely, seeding from the lymphatic circulation.

Direct extension from calvarial metastasis is more common in lung, prostate, breast carcinomas and Ewing sarcomas [2, 6]. When calvarial lesions are not present hematogenous seeding is a possible explanation. Sgouros et al., reported a combination of cutaneous metastasis in the scalp of the occiput with ipsilateral dural metastasis in the posterior fossa, on the inferior surface of the tentorium suggesting spread via the external carotid artery [17]. Another piece of evidence supporting the role of arterial route is that it is often a concomitant finding with brain metastasis and lung disease especially in the presence of lymphangitic and intravascular pulmonary invasion [2]. Dissemination via Batson's plexus has been postulated to occur in prostate cancer explaining the high frequency of skull and dural metastasis with this tumor [2, 18, 19].

Clinical Findings

Symptoms from dural metastasis are usually related to compression or invasion of underlying brain, production of subdural hematomas [20–26] or fluid collections and less often by obstruction of blood flow in the venous sinuses. About 20% of patients with DM are asymptomatic and DM is fortuitously identified during a radiological work-up or necropsy.

Symptoms related to compression or invasion of underlying brain are typically indicative of intracranial hypertension with headaches, progressive motor deficits, sensory deficits, mental status changes, speech impairment, cranial neuropathy and seizures (table 2) [1, 27](Figure 1) Dural metastases, although rare, are the leading cause of sinus thrombosis in patients with solid tumors, producing symptoms of intracranial hypertension [28, 29].

Non-traumatic subdural hematoma resulting from neoplastic invasion of the meninges, or pachymeningitis carcinomatosa is a classic complication of dural seeding, with an incidence ranging from 15–40% [2]. Minette et al., in a series of

Table 2. Adapted from reference [2]

Symptoms and Signs in 89 patients with dural metastasis
Elevated intracranial pressure (23.5%)
Neurological deficits (20%)
Coma (10%)
Cranial neuropathy (10%)
Seizure (9%)
Headache (7%)
Confusion (4.5%)
No symptom (16%)

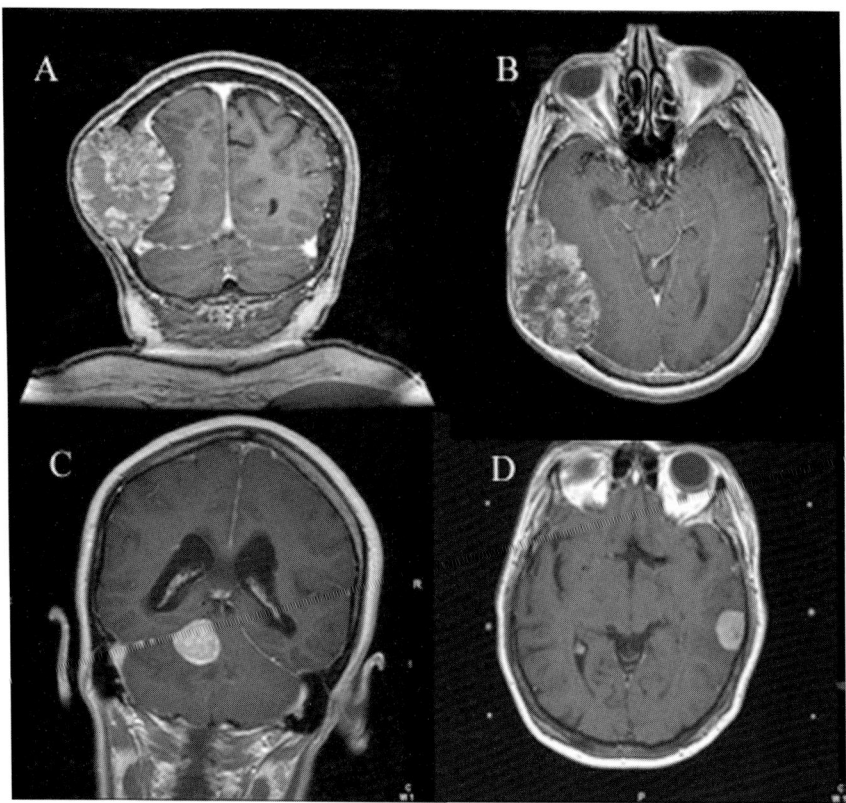

Figure 1. (**A**) Coronal-T1 with contrast, and (**B**) Axial-T1 with contrast MRI of a 70 year-old woman with metastatic adenocarcinoma of the dura and bone with compression of the underlying brain. (**C**) Coronal-T1 with contrast MRI of a right tentorial metastatic adenocarcinoma favoring lung primary, clinically interpreted as a meningioma. (**D**)Axial-T1 with contrast MRI of a 45 year-old woman with metastatic breast adenocarcinoma to the left temporal dura. Courtesy of Dr. Mark Shaffrey, Department of Neurosurgery, University of Virginia.

70 patients with subdural hematomas and systemic cancer, found dural metastatic involvement as the primary cause in 2 among 10 patients with solid tumors and in 6 among 28 patients with hematologic malignancies [30]. The authors also acknowledge that microscopic inspection of the dura either at operation or at autopsy was not performed in all cases which may have underestimated the actual incidence of dural metastatic lesions [30]. Kunii et al. in a literature review found adenocarcinomas to be the most common metastatic tumor associated with subdural hematomas [31]. Several hypotheses have been postulated to explain that tendency

of the dura to form subdural collections. Firstly, fragile tumor neo-vessels may rupture within the subdural space [32, 33]. Secondly, obstruction of the dural veins by tumor cells may cause dilation of the capillaries in the inner areolar layer, followed by rupture and subdural bleeding [18, 34–36]. The third mechanism proposed by Chen et al. would consider the subdural hematoma as mediator of subdural invasion of tumor cells which would otherwise be barred from the subdural space: the process of subdural membrane formation with neovascularization in both the membrane and dura may alter the barrier characteristics of the dura mater in a way that allows either direct or hematogenous spread of tumor cells across the dural membrane. After the membranes have been seeded, they become hypervascular or increasingly fragile, which may account for multiple repeated hemorrhages within the subdural compartment resulting in septations of the loculations of varying ages [37].

A case of extradural hematoma in a patient who was later found to have dural metastases secondary to bronchogenic carcinoma was reported by Shamim et al. [38].

Diagnosis

The radiological diagnosis of DM relies upon CT scans and MR images (Figure 1). CT scans, although less reliable than MRI for the assessment of the extent of intracranial lesions, offer the ability to detect bone involvement on bone windows [39]. MR images provides better contrast resolution, multiplanar imaging, ability to detect incipient dural seeding; MRI is the only technique capable of depicting dural metastases as enhancing dural masses extending along bone structures [40]. The classic MR imaging suggestive of DM is a homogeneous contrast-enhancing mass with increased signal on T2-weighted images, thickening of the dura mater, and an enhancing dural tail that can be suggestive of a meningioma [41].

The main differential diagnosis of a DM is meningioma, and several reports have addressed this issue [9, 41–46]. Laigle-Donadey et al. found 23 cases among the 198 cases of dural metastasis in their literature review where a meningioma was considered in the differential diagnosis, particularly in patients with prostate cancer where the osteoblastic pattern of bony lesions appears as hyperostosis [2]. Well-known radiological features of a meningioma, usually a well circumscribed, extra-axial, hyperdense, contrast-enhancing lesion, sometimes with osteoblastic reaction can be found in dural metastasis from different primary sites [42] (Figure 1). The "dural tail sign" seen on MRI which was considered highly suggestive of a meningioma, can also be observed in dural metastasis [47, 48].

Advanced MR techniques play an important role in helping to differentiate DMs from meningiomas. Bendszus et al., using MR spectroscopy found a high lipid signal exclusively in metastasis consistent with necrosis, which is not exclusive but highly suggestive of a malignant lesion [48]. Kremer et al., using conventional MR imaging suggested that low rCBV (relative cerebral blood volume) may be indicative of metastasis over meningiomas [49]. Nathoo et al., suggested that the use of 111-indium-octreotide brain scintigraphy together with FDG-PET scanning, may be useful to increase diagnostic specificity of conventional MRI in the differential diagnosis between meningiomas and other dural-based pathologies [50].

Treatment

Treatment usually consists in surgical resection when there is a single, well-circumscribed and surgically accessible lesion with reasonably controlled extracranial disease. In patients with progressive systemic disease but with life-threatening lesions causing symptoms related to intracranial hypertension, surgical resection is recommended. In patients presenting with subdural hematomas, immediate evacuation can be life-saving, and especially in those patients known to have primary systemic disease, dural sampling and cytologic analysis of the fluid drained can be diagnostic [1, 51, 52].

High-dose of glucocorticoids (dexamethasone) may produce transitory symptomatic relief even if there is no evidence of cerebral edema [2, 10].

In Laigle-Donadey's literature review, 83% of the patients underwent surgery alone or associated with another treatment, and the authors concluded that this number overestimates the number of patients eligible for surgery, and is probably biased by a high number of surgical series [2].

Radiation therapy can be used to palliate dural metastasis, either whole brain radiation therapy (WBRT) if the dural lesion is accompanied by parenchymal metastasis or stereotactic radiosurgery (SRS) for isolated lesions less than 3 cm in diameter [53–56].

The benefits of chemotherapy have not been clearly demonstrated for patients with brain metastasis. Consequently, chemotherapy should be reserved for patients who have failed radiation therapy or those who have chemosensitive tumors such as lymphomas and germ cell tumors [57].

Prognosis

The prognosis for dural metastasis may be extrapolated from the prognosis of brain metastasis in general and remains less than 1 year, with most patients dying from systemic disease rather than direct neurological complications [57]. Recursive partitioning analysis (RPA) in patients with brain metastasis, yielded factors that might predict overall survival such as: KPS > 70, age < 65, controlled primary tumor, and absence of extracranial metastasis [58]. More favorable courses were principally observed in hematological cancers, breast and prostate carcinomas with a median survival of 365, 273, and 120 days respectively, as reported in Laigle-Donadey's review [2].

Skull Base Metastasis

Introduction

The skull base encompasses the ethmoid and sphenoid bones, and the basal parts of the frontal, temporal, and occipital bones. Within the skull base there are several foramina where the cranial nerves and vessels enter and exit the skull; therefore neoplasms of the skull base will likely cause early symptoms due to cranial nerve dysfunction. Skull base infiltration by direct extension of primary head and neck tumors is not the object of this chapter.

The incidence of skull base metastasis is probably underestimated in studies based on hospital records and death certificates, since many patients may not exhibit the classic signs and symptoms of skull base metastasis. Furthermore the skull base is not often explored during autopsy [59]. The most frequent metastatic tumors to the skull base are breast, lung, and prostate, followed by renal, thyroid, and melanoma [59]. Greenberg et al., in a retrospective series of 43 patients found breast, lung, and prostate accounting respectively for 40, 14, and 12% of the cases [60].Laigle-Donadey et al., in a literature review of the English and French literature between 1963 and 2003, found 279 cases of skull base metastasis, with prostate, breast, lymphoma, and lung responsible for 38.5, 20.5, 8, and 6% of the cases [61]. Skull base metastases are often a late event in the natural history of cancer and many patients already have disseminated disease including other bone metastases [60, 62]. However, skull base involvement can be the first sign of cancer, as was observed in 28% of the patients in Laigle-Donadey series [61]

Pathophysiology

Direct hematogenous spread most likely accounts for the majority of skull base metastasis. Blood-borne emboli reach the basal cranium through small anastomotic arteries at the neural foramina [63]. Another possible mechanism advocated especially in prostate cancer is retrograde seeding through the valveless Batson's venous plexus [64, 65]. With increased intra-abdominal and intra-thoracic pressure, blood is shunted through the valveless vertebral, prevertebral, and epidural veins to reach the basilar plexus of veins, which is continuous with the venous plexi of the basicranium, without traversing the lungs [19, 63, 66].

Clinical Findings

Cranial neuropathies secondary to a skull base metastasis may be the first clinical manifestation of a distant cancer [67, 68], and they can be clinically silent until their growth produces pain or cranial nerves palsies [69].

Clinical manifestations depend upon the location of the metastasis, resulting in pain and/or involvement of a single or multiple cranial nerves.

Greenberg et al., retrospectively studying 43 patients with skull base metastasis, identified five different clinical syndromes: orbital syndrome (7%), parasellar syndrome (16%), middle fossa syndrome (35%), jugular foramen syndrome (16 %), and occipital condyle syndrome (21%) [60]. Laigle-Donadey et al., found a predominance of the parasellar and sellar syndromes (29%), middle-fossa syndrome (6%), and jugular foramen syndrome (3.5%); however in one-third of their cases a specific syndrome could not be identified [61].

The clinical findings in skull base metastasis are summarized in table 3.

Orbital Syndrome

The orbit is an unusual site of dissemination for systemic cancers, accounting for between 2–10% of skull base metastases [60, 70]. Font et al. reported 28 cases of pure orbital involvement among 227 cases of carcinomas metastatic to the eye and orbit [71]. Rarely a pure orbital syndrome is found. Laigle-Donadey found orbital

Table 3. Clinical finding in skull base metastases. Adapted from references[60, 61, 63]

Syndrome	Neural Structures	Clinical Findings
Orbital	Extraocular muscles CNs III, IV, VI, and V1	Supraorbital or/and orbital painOphthalmoplegia (diplopia) Facial numbness (V1) Decreased visionPeriorbital swelling/tenderness.
Parasellar	CNs III, IV, VI, and V1	Frontal headache (unilateral) Ophthalmoplegia (diplopia) Facial numbness (V1) Periorbital swelling.
Gasserian ganglion	CN V (mainly V2, V3), sensory and motor. Remotely, III, IV, VI, and VII.	Facial numbness (V2, V3) Unilateral pterygoid and/or masseter weakness. Abducens palsy (anterior ridge) Facial palsy (posterior ridge).
Temporal bone	Middle ear CNs VII and VIII	Hearing loss Otalgia Periauricular swelling Facial palsy.
Jugular foramen	CNs IX, X, XI, and XII	Occipital/postauricular pain (unilateral) Dysphagia Hoarseness Weakness of palate, vocal cord paralysis, SCM/trapezius atrophy, tongue atrophy and Horner's syndrome.
Occipital condyle	CN XII	Occipital pain Neck stiffness/pain Dysarthria/ Dysphagia Ipsilateral tongue weakness.
Numb chin syndrome	Mental nerve over the chin and lower lip.	Unilateral anesthesia of the chin and lower lip.

SCM = sternocleidomastoid muscle.

metastasis most frequently due to prostate carcinoma (56%), lymphoma (23%), and breast carcinoma (15%) [61]. Greenberg et al. found metastasis to the orbit in only 3 patients (7%) in his series [60].

The orbital syndrome is characterized by frontal headache usually described as a progressive, dull, continuous pain in the supraorbital area over the affected eye, red eye, peri-orbital swelling and tenderness, and proptosis, associated with diplopia, which is often preceded by blurred binocular vision [70–74]. Proptosis along with some degree of ophthalmoplegia is the most common finding in orbital syndrome after pain [62]. A palpable mass inside the orbit may be present and is easily detected clinically. Sensory loss over the territory of the ophthalmic division of the trigeminal nerve (V1), can be also found [60]. Decreased vision, visual field cuts, and papilledema rarely occur until very late in the disease course: this may happen because tumors grow into the orbit from bone, preserving the optic nerve where the muscle cone is located [60, 63]. Enophthalmos has been reported in patients with scirrhous carcinoma of the breast [71, 75].

Parasellar Syndrome

Parasellar or sphenocavernous sinus metastasis are also uncommon, with reports indicating an incidence less than 7% of all mass lesions in this area [76, 77] (Figure 2A,B). If considered together with sellar metastasis, the frequency may increase to up to 29% in one review [61]. Roessmann et al. reported 16 (27%) parasellar lesions in 60 patients with carcinoma at autopsy, and 9 of them the primary tumor was breast cancer [78]. Metastatic systemic lymphomas seem to have a predilection for the cavernous sinus region; therefore, a cavernous sinus syndrome combined with visual loss may be the first manifestation of a systemic lymphoma [61, 79].

The parasellar syndrome usually results from metastasis to either the petrous apex or the sella turcica with contiguous extension to the cavernous sinus. It is usually unilateral but there are reports of bilateral cavernous sinus involvement [80]. The syndrome consists of ophthalmoplegia as a result of damage to the oculomotor nerves (III, IV, and VI), and oculosympathetic nerves as they travel thru the cavernous sinus, and also facial pain, dysesthesia, and paraesthesia caused by damage to one or more of the divisions of the trigeminal nerve, traveling in the dural wall of the cavernous sinus [81–83]. Headaches may be present as an initial symptom in 83% of the cases [60].

Clinical examination shows various degrees of ophthalmoplegia and facial numbness, associated or not with periorbital swelling [84].

Middle Fossa (Gasserian Ganglion Syndrome)

The middle fossa syndrome is characterized by numbness, paresthesias, and/or pain referred to the trigeminal nerve distribution, usually sparing the frontal region. The

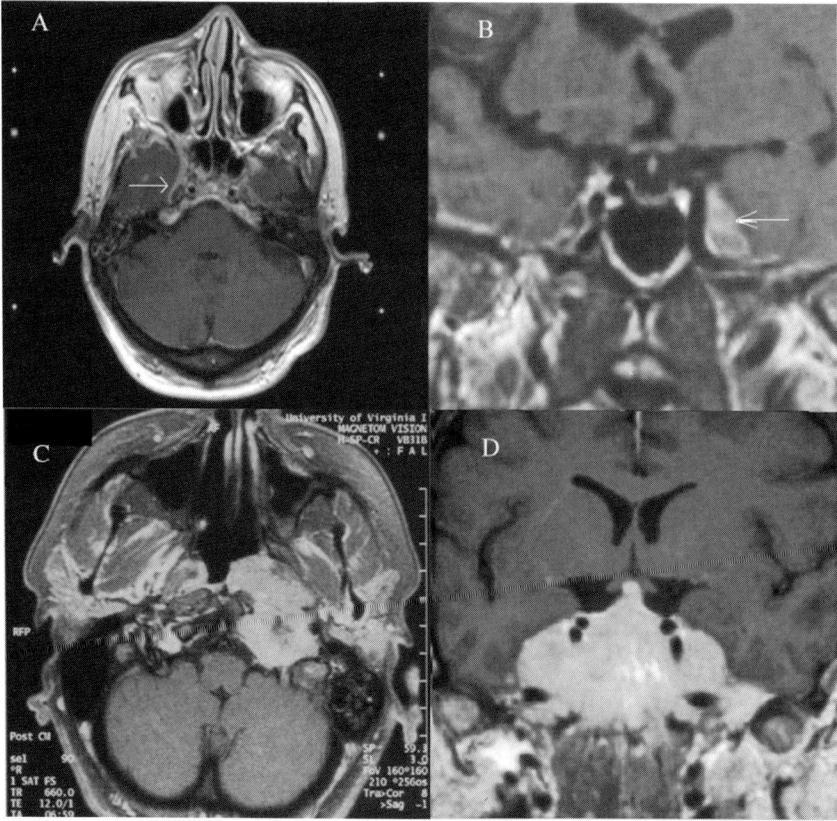

Figure 2. (A)Axial-T1 with contrast MRI of an adenoid cystic carcinoma metastatic to the right cavernous sinus (arrow). **(B)** Coronal-T1 with contrast MRI of a squamous cell carcinoma metastatic to the left cavernous sinus (courtesy of Dr. Maurice Lipper, University of Virginia). **(C)** Axial-T1 with contrast MRI of a breast adenocarcinoma metastatic to the skull base. The lesion is located on the left clivus invading the pre-vertebral space, hypoglossal canal and bulging into the nasopharynx. Courtesy of Dr. C. Douglas Phillips, University of Virginia. **(D)** Coronal-T1 with contrast MRI of a plasmacytoma invading the sellar and parasellar compartment. Courtesy of Dr. Maurice Lipper, University of Virginia.

pain is often "lightning-like" similar to an idiopathic trigeminal neuralgia. Some patients can manifest involvement of the motor root of the trigeminal nerve [61]. Headache was reported in 23% of the patients with middle fossa syndrome in the Memorial Sloan-Kettering series, in marked contrast to the parasellar syndrome, in which 83% presented headache as an initial symptom [60]. Twenty per cent of patients with middle fossa metastasis had diplopia due to abducens palsy probably by nerve compression in Dorello's canal, and 26% had other oculomotor nerve palsy that may have been related to medial extension of the tumor into the parasellar area [60]. Tumor spread along the posterior ridge of the petrous bone may also compress the facial nerve [63, 85]. Several reports suggest that breast cancer is the most common skull base systemic metastasis causing middle fossa syndrome [60, 86, 87], but lung cancer has also been reported [88].

Jugular Foramen Syndrome

Metastatic spread to the jugular foramen and the adjacent hypoglossal canal may result in Collet-Sicard syndrome, consisting of paralysis of the lower four cranial nerves (XI, X, XI, and XII), and in different combination of paralysis of these nerves, also classically recalled by eponyms: paralysis of IX, X, and XI (Vernet syndrome), paralysis of the lower four cranial nerves accompanied by ipsilateral Horner's syndrome (Villaret syndrome) [89, 90] (Figure 2C).

Clinically patients may present with unilateral occipital or postauricular pain, hoarseness, and dysphagia. Signs may include palate weakness, vocal cord paralysis, weakness and atrophy of the ipsilateral sternocleidomastoid muscle and the upper part of the trapezius, and occasionally Horner's syndrome. When the hypoglossal nerve is affected, ipsilateral weakness and atrophy of the tongue may be present. Rarely glossopharyngeal neuralgia is found, and a case of jugular foramen syndrome presenting with papilledema, probably due to obstruction of the transverse sinus, has been described [91]. Different types of systemic cancers causing spreading to the jugular foramen, causing Collet-Sicard syndrome and other patterns of cranial nerve paralysis such as breast [92], melanoma [93], Ewing's sarcoma [91], and prostate [89, 90, 94, 95], have been reported.

Temporal Bone Syndrome

The most common manifestation of temporal bone metastasis is conductive hearing loss, present in approximately 30–40% of patients. It is almost always the result of dysfunction of the Eustachian tube with secondary serous otitis media [96–98]. Sensorineural hearing loss may occur due to the involvement of the cochlear fibers in the internal auditory meatus [85]. Otorrhea, vertigo, tinnitus, and middle ear effusion are rarely found [96].

Facial nerve paralysis caused by skull base metastasis has been often reported in the literature [99–104]. Jung et al. in a study of 60 temporal bones with metastatic disease, found involvement of the facial nerve in 14 (23%) [105]. One study pointed out that only 50% of patients with tumoral invasion of the facial canal clinically had some degree of facial paralysis, although virtually all patients with tumor extension beyond the epineural sheath had complete paralysis [99]. Schuknecht et al. also reported a high incidence of facial palsy [106]. Maddox et al. emphasized that the triad of otalgia, periauricular swelling, and facial nerve paralysis in a patient with systemic cancer is highly suspicious for metastatic spread to the temporal bone

[85]. Breast, lung, and prostate cancers in this order are the most common etiology of temporal bone metastasis [96].

Occipital Condyle Syndrome

Occipital condyle syndrome consists of unilateral occipital region pain associated with ipsilateral XIIth nerve palsy that usually occurs a few weeks later [107, 108, 109]. Patients frequently complain of severe, continuous, unilateral occipital region pain, typically exacerbated by neck flexion and rotation of the head to the side contralateral to the pain. The pain can radiate anteriorly to the forehead in some patients and is often associated with stiff neck [108, 110, 111]. Along the course of the disease virtually all patients develop dysarthria and dysphagia related to difficulties moving the tongue. The involvement of the hypoglossal nerve is often unilateral [108, 112, 113], but bilateral involvement can occur[114].

On examination, there is tenderness to palpation over the occipital area and ipsilateral tongue weakness, atrophy and sometimes fasciculation [107].

Seven out of nine patients with occipital condyle syndrome in Greenberg's series had the typical occipital pain, four had dysarthria, two had dysphagia, and all had ipsilateral tongue weakness [60]. Breast cancer in women and prostate cancer in men are the most common malignancies spreading to the occipital condyle [107].

Numb Chin Syndrome (NCS)

The NCS, also known as mental neuropathy, is characterized by numbness in the area supplied by the mental nerve and is a rare manifestation of metastatic cancer [115]. It is a pure sensory neuropathy because the inferior alveolar nerve has no motor fibers [116]. Chin numbness is caused by malignant infiltration of the inferior alveolar nerve sheet or compression of the nerve by jaw metastasis or local tumor [117]. Intracranial involvement of the mandibular nerve by lesion at the skull base has also been reported [118].

NCS is associated with neoplastic processes, in particular breast cancer and lymphomas [119–121], but other types of cancers including melanoma [122], lung [115], prostate [123], have been reported to cause NCS. Physicians and dentists should consider metastatic cancer in patients who present with chin numbness without obvious cause for their complaint.

Sellar Syndrome

Metastases to the pituitary gland causing pituitary dysfunction, has been well described in the literature from various types of systemic cancer [124, 125] (Figure 2D).

The most common presentation of a pituitary metastasis is diabetes insipidus, reflecting the predominance of metastases to the posterior lobe of the hypophysis [126]. McCormick et al. reviewing 40 symptomatic cases, noted diabetes insipidus in 70%, and only 15% of the patients had one or more pituitary deficiencies [127]. However, recent studies using more sensitive imaging techniques and endocrinological tests have increased the incidence of anterior lobe involvement [128, 129]. Morita et al. reported hypothyroidism and hypoadrenalism as to be the most common signs of symptomatic hypopituitarism, followed by hypogonadism [129].

The most important criteria to differentiate pituitary metastases from adenomas seem to be diabetes insipidus. Diabetes insipidus is present in only 1% of pituitary adenomas [126, 130]. Sometimes when the metastasis spreads laterally there may be an associated parasellar syndrome. Breast and lung cancer are the most common primary neoplasm metastasizing to the pituitary [126, 131]. Sudden onset of diabetes insipidus, ophthalmoplegia, and headaches in a patient over 50 yr old should raise the suspicion of pituitary metastases, regardless of a history of malignancy.

Diagnosis

The majority of skull base tumors produce lytic lesions, with the exception of prostate and lung cancers that can produce either lytic or osteoblastic lesions [132]. Thus, although plain X-rays of the skull base may show some evidence of bone erosion, they are low yield studies because of difficulties in their interpretation.

Computed tomography (CT) and magnetic resonance imaging (MRI) have long been the mainstay of the diagnosis of skull base lesions [133]. Preoperative imaging can define the extent of tumor, suggest the best surgical approach, assess the involvement of critical structures, and identify pathologic entities that have a characteristic imaging profile [133–135].

CT scans with bone windows are the best method to show bone lesions whose aspect is lytic and MRI is superior for detection of a contrast enhancing soft tissue mass [61, 136]. New CT scanners with 3-D reconstructions provide soft tissue and bony detail with very high resolutions for small structures such as the neural foramina [135]. CT angiography can be used to assess vascular structures noninvasively, and CT perfusion may be useful to differentiate between malignant and benign tumors [133].

Advances in MRI sequences have allowed high-resolution imaging of labyrinthine structures, cranial nerves, perineural tumor spread, cavernous sinus invasion, and vascular abnormalities using MR angiography and MR venography [133]. Perineural tumor spread can be studied using magnetization-prepared rapid gradient echo (MP-RAGE) [137]. MP-RAGE and T1-weighted images with fat saturation are useful to detect dural invasion by tumor, the dura appears thickened and enhances intensely [138].

Radionuclide scans are useful to detect bone metastasis, their sensitivity to detect skull base lesions is around 30–50% in patients whose radiographic studies was normal [139]. The major setback of radionuclide studies is the increased activity associated with conditions such as sinusitis, mastoiditis, or temporomandibular joint arthrosis.

SPECT scans may be helpful to diagnose skull base deposits, especially when they show a focus of abnormal uptake of 99mTc-HMDP in the skull base that corroborates the clinical findings [140].

PET scan and PET/CT scan are useful for initial staging of skull base tumors but will increasingly be the mainstay of response to therapy and detection of recurrent disease [133, 141].

CSF examination is particular useful to exclude meningeal carcinomatosis [61].In patients with multiple cranial neuropathies whose CT and MRI are inconclusive and the spinal fluid is normal, skull base metastasis becomes the most likely diagnosis [63].

Treatment

Treatment of skull base metastases may require a combination of surgery, radiation therapy, and chemotherapy, with the latter two being the mainstays of therapy. Surgery is obviously only appropriate for patients with solitary metastasis without active extracranial disease, which significantly reduces the number of surgical candidates (Figure 3). Advances in techniques for primary skull base tumors make the resection of solitary skull base metastasis possible [142–145]. Metastasis in the sellar and parasellar regions are more suitable to surgical treatment, either via craniotomy or transphenoidal route [76]. Jia et al. reported a series of 15 patients with skull base metastasis, 7 of them located in the anterior skull base in which total resection was accomplished in 13 and subtotal resection in 2. CSF leakage was the main complication found [146].

Hanbali et al. reported 12 cases that have undergone resection for skull base metastasis at M.D. Anderson, among 439 other skull base tumor resections (2.7%), between November 1992 and August 2002 [147]. In four patients the diagnosis was renal cell carcinoma. Six patients (50%) had local tumor recurrence with the mean time to recurrence being only 4.3 months, and the other six patients remained free of recurrence at a mean time of 14.3 months. The authors noted a poor outcome for patients with malignant epithelial tumors such as renal cell carcinoma and melanoma: the exception may be patients with follicular carcinoma of the thyroid for whom effective post surgical therapies are available like radioactive iodine and thyroid suppression.

Radiation therapy appears to be the standard treatment for skull base metastasis, with significant pain relief and improvement of neurological deficits. The rate of neurological improvement after radiation therapy appears to be closely related to the precocity of the treatment after the onset of the symptoms. Vikram et al. reported 46 cases of skull base metastasis treated with radiation therapy and observed that 87% of the patients improved after treatment if symptoms were present for less than

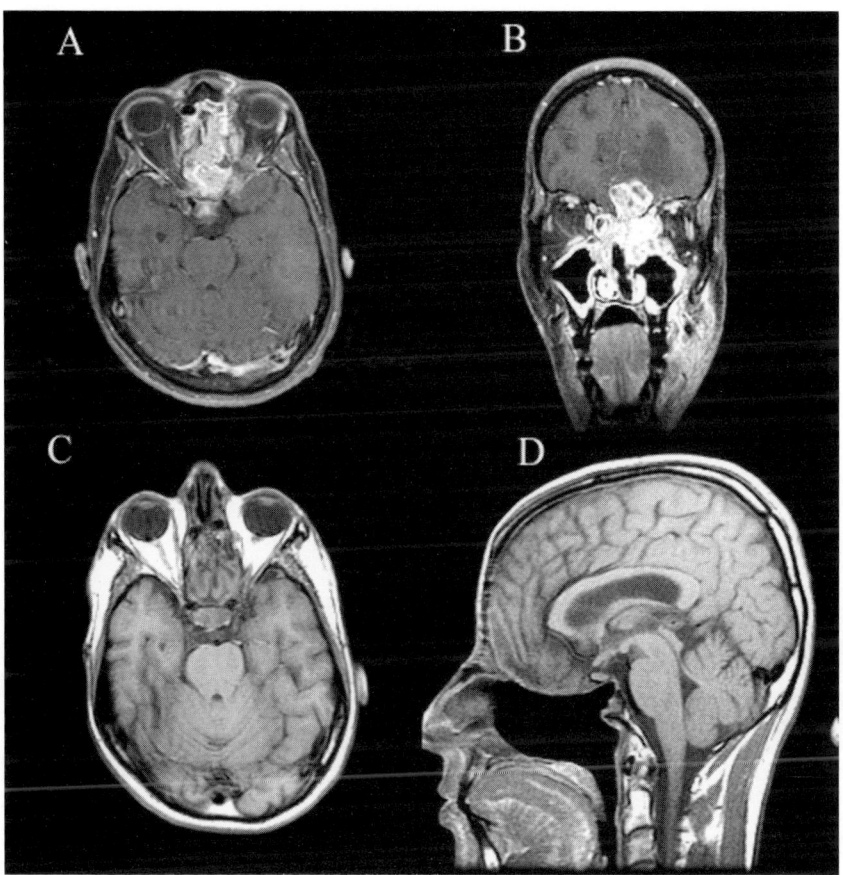

Figure 3. (A)Pre-operative axial-T1, and (**B**) coronal-T1 with contrast MRI of a 30 year-old man with an ethmoidal squamous-cell carcinoma. (**C**) Post-operative axial-T1, and (**D**) Post-operative axial-T1 with contrast MRI showing gross total resection of the lesion. Courtesy of Dr. Daniel Prevedello and Dr. Amin Kassam, Department of Neurosurgery, University of Pittsburgh.

1 month. On the other hand, only 25% improved if the symptoms were present for 3 months or more [148]. Another smaller series of 13 patients reported complete or almost complete restoration of cranial nerve function in 8 patients, using different radiation therapy dosages and techniques [149]. The radiation therapy schedule is usually 30Gy in 10 days over 2 weeks given that these patients generally have poor overall survival and this fractionation regimen is habitually well tolerated with a small risk of long-term sequelae. In patients with controlled systemic disease and long-term life expectancy, 50Gy with 1.8 or 2Gy per fraction is reasonable. Response to radiation therapy reflects the radiosensitivity profile of the primary

tumor; therefore, patients with lymphoma and breast cancer have a better response to smaller doses of radiation than patients with prostate or lung cancer [61, 150].

In addition to conventional radiation therapy there are several reports in the literature supporting the use of stereotactic radiosurgery or fractionated stereotactic radiation therapy in the treatment of skull base metastases [151–156]. Stereotactic radiosurgery using either Gamma-Knife or Linac based systems is able to deliver a large dose of radiation in a single fraction and fractionated stereotactic radiation therapy is able to deliver large doses in multiple smaller fractions. These techniques have the advantage of being very conformal and they can be used in patients previously treated with conventional radiation therapy for head and neck cancers who developed recurrence or metastases at the skull base.

Iwai et al. reported a series of 21 patients with cavernous sinus metastasis and invasion treated with Gamma-Knife radiosurgery [155]. Twelve patients had metastases from distant sites and 9 had nasopharyngeal carcinoma, clinical improvement was achieved in 48% of the patients and tumor growth control was observed in 67% at their final follow-up. Francel et al. published the results of 71 patients treated with Gamma-Knife radiosurgery and with a follow-up of 1 year or more, the tumor was smaller in 34% and unchanged or smaller in 93%[151].

These results suggest that stereotactic radiosurgery provides good local control and complication rates comparable to standard radiation therapy and it can be reliably used mainly in patients with lesions near neural structures or in previously irradiated fields.

Prognosis

The prognosis of patients with skull base metastases also largely depends upon the histological diagnosis of the primary tumor, systemic control, site, and size of the lesion. Cranial nerve palsies have been reported to indicate a poorer prognosis with an average survival of 5 months after the onset of cranial nerve involvement; however some cases of prostate cancer have been reported as exceptions [84, 150, 157, 158]. In Long-Donadey's literature review the overall median survival was 31 months, with breast carcinomas associated with better outcomes [61].

References

1. Posner J. Intracranial metastasis. In: Posner J, eds. Neurologic Complications of Cancer. F.A. Davis, Philadelphia., 1995:77–110.
2. Laigle-Donadey F, Taillibert S, Mokhtari K, Hildebrand J and Delattre JY. Dural metastases. J Neurooncol 2005;75(1):57–61.
3. Meyer PC, Reath TG. Secondary neoplasms of the central nervous system and meninges. Br J Cancer 1953;7(4):438–48.

4. Lesse S, Netsky MG. Metastasis of neoplasms to the central nervous system and meninges. AMA Arch Neurol Psychiatry 1954;72(2):133–53.
5. Posner JB, Chernik NL. Intracranial metastases from systemic cancer. In: Schoenberg BS, eds. Advances in Neurology. New York, NY: Raven Press, 1978:579–592.
6. Kleinschmidt-DeMasters BK. Dural metastases. A retrospective surgical and autopsy series. Arch Pathol Lab Med 2001;125(7):880–7.
7. France LH. Contribution to the study of 150 cases of cerebral metastases. II. Neuropathological study. J Neurosurg Sci 1975;19(4):189–210.
8. Takakura K, Sano K, Hojo S and Hirano A. Metastatic Tumors of the Central Nervous System. Tokio, Japan: Igaku-Shoin Ltd, 1982.
9. Ahn JY, Kim NK, Oh D and Ahn HJ. Thymic carcinoma with brain metastasis mimicking meningioma. J Neurooncol 2002;58(3):193–9.
10. Bentley AM, Keen JC. Dural metastases in prostate cancer. Clin Oncol (R Coll Radiol) 2003;15(3):165–6.
11. Higuchi M, Fujimoto Y, Miyahara E and Ikeda H. Isolated dural metastasis from colon cancer. Clin Neurol Neurosurg 1997;99(2):135–7.
12. Maezawa H. Dural metastasis of prostatic carcinoma on the middle fossa. No To Shinkei 1998;50(11):1034–5.
13. Maiuri F, Esposito F, Del Basso De Caro,M. and Tortora F. Dural cerebellopontine angle metastasis from malignant parotid oncocytoma. J Neurooncol 2003;61(1):69–72.
14. Oyoshi T, Nakayama M, Hirano H, Shimokawa S and Kuratsu J. Intracranial dural metastasis of mediastinal seminoma–case report. Neurol Med Chir (Tokyo) 2000;40(8):423–6.
15. Tsukada Y, Fouad A, Pickren JW and Lane WW. Central nervous system metastasis from breast carcinoma. Autopsy study. Cancer 1983;52(12):2349–54.
16. Scarrow AM, Rajendran PR and Marion D. Metastatic prostate adenocarcinoma of the dura mater. Br J Neurosurg 2000;14(5):473–4.
17. Sgouros S, Walsh AR. Synchronous dural and cutaneous metastases along the distribution of the external carotid artery. Br J Neurosurg 1994;8(5):617–9.
18. Cobo Dols M, Gil Calle S and Villar Chamorro E, et al. Dural metastases with subdural hematoma from prostate cancer. Oncologia 2005;28(8):407–11.
19. Batson OV. The vertebral system of veins as a means for cancer dissemination. Prog Clin Cancer 1967;3:1–18.
20. Tomlin JM, Alleyne CH. Transdural metastasis from adenocarcinoma of the prostate mimicking subdural hematoma: case report. Surg Neurol 2002;58(5):329,31; discussion 331.
21. McKenzie CR, Rengachary SS, McGregor DH, Dixon AY and Suskind DL. Subdural hematoma associated with metastatic neoplasms. Neurosurgery 1990;27(4):619,24; discussion 624–5.

93. Schweinfurth JM, Johnson JT and Weissman J. Jugular foramen syndrome as a complication of metastatic melanoma. Am J Otolaryngol 1993;14(3):168–74.

94. Chacon G, Alexandraki I and Palacio C. Collet-sicard syndrome: an uncommon manifestation of metastatic prostate cancer. South Med J 2006;99(8):898–9.

95. Satoh H, Nishiyama T, Horiguchi A, Nakashima J, Saito S and Murai M. A case of Collet-Sicard syndrome caused by skull base metastasis of prostate carcinoma. Nippon Hinyokika Gakkai Zasshi 2000;91(6):562–4.

96. Gloria-Cruz TI, Schachern PA, Paparella MM, Adams GL and Fulton SE. Metastases to temporal bones from primary nonsystemic malignant neoplasms. Arch Otolaryngol Head Neck Surg 2000;126(2):209–14.

97. Berlinger NT, Koutroupas S, Adams G and Maisel R. Patterns of involvement of the temporal bone in metastatic and systemic malignancy. Laryngoscope 1980;90(4):619–27.

98. Saldanha CB, Bennett JD, Evans JN and Pambakian H. Metastasis to the temporal bone, secondary to carcinoma of the bladder. J Laryngol Otol 1989;103(6):599–601.

99. Saito H, Chinzei K and Furuta M. Pathological features of peripheral facial paralysis caused by malignant tumour. Acta Otolaryngol Suppl 1988;446: 165–71.

100. Miro Castillo N, Roca-Ribas Serda F, Barnadas Molins A, Prades Marti J, Casamitjana Claramunt F and Perello Scherdel E. Facial paralysis of metastatic origin. Review of metastatic lesions of the temporal bone. An Otorrinolaringol Ibero Am 2000;27(3):255–63.

101. Nagai M, Yamada H and Kitamoto M, et al. Facial nerve palsy due to temporal bone metastasis from hepatocellular carcinoma. J Gastroenterol Hepatol 2005;20(7):1131–2.

102. Weiss MD, Kattah JC, Jones R and Manz HJ. Isolated facial nerve palsy from metastasis to the temporal bone: report of two cases and a review of the literature. Am J Clin Oncol 1997;20(1):19–23.

103. Marzo SJ, Leonetti JP and Petruzzelli G. Facial paralysis caused by malignant skull base neoplasms. Neurosurg Focus 2002;12(5):e2.

104. Lan MY, Shiao AS and Li WY. Facial paralysis caused by metastasis of breast carcinoma to the temporal bone. J Chin Med Assoc 2004;67(11):587–90.

105. Jung TT, Jun BH, Shea D and Paparella MM. Primary and secondary tumors of the facial nerve. A temporal bone study. Arch Otolaryngol Head Neck Surg 1986;112(12):1269–73.

106. Schuknecht HF, Allam AF and Murakami Y. Pathology of secondary malignant tumors of the temporal bone. Ann Otol Rhinol Laryngol 1968;77(1):5–22.

107. Capobianco DJ, Brazis PW, Rubino FA and Dalton JN. Occipital condyle syndrome. Headache 2002;42(2):142–6.

108. Combarros O, Alvarez de Arcaya A and Berciano J. Isolated unilateral hypoglossal nerve palsy: nine cases. J Neurol 1998;245(2):98–100.

109. Endo K, Okano R, Kuroda Y, Yamada S and Tabei K. Renal cell carcinoma with skull base metastasis preceded by paraneoplastic signs in a chronic hemodialysis patient. Intern Med 2001;40(9):924–30.

110. Moris G, Roig C, Misiego M, Alvarez A, Berciano J and Pascual J. The distinctive headache of the occipital condyle syndrome: a report of four cases. Headache 1998;38(4):308–11.

111. Pascual J, Gutierrez A, Polo JM and Berciano J. Occipital condyle syndrome: presentation of a case. Neurologia 1989;4(8):293–5.

112. Pavithran K, Doval DC, Hukku S and Jena A. Isolated hypoglossal nerve palsy due to skull base metastasis from breast cancer. Australas Radiol 2001;45(4):534–5.

113. Romero M, Paradas C and Torrecilla MD. Isolated paralysis of the hypoglossal nerve due to metastasis at the base of the cranium. Neurologia 2000;15(1):31.

114. Rotta FT, Romano JG. Skull base metastases causing acute bilateral hypoglossal nerve palsy. J Neurol Sci 1997;148(1):127–9.

115. Marinella MA. Metastatic large cell lung cancer presenting with numb chin syndrome. Respir Med 1997;91(4):235–6.

116. Kapa Baskaran R, Ramanarayanan K and Smith M. Numb Chin Syndrome-A reflection of systemic malignancy. World J Surg Oncol 2006;4(1):52.

117. Laurencet FM, Anchisi S, Tullen E and Dietrich PY. Mental neuropathy: report of five cases and review of the literature. Crit Rev Oncol Hematol 2000;34(1):71–9.

118. Burt RK, Sharfman WH, Karp BI and Wilson WH. Mental neuropathy (numb chin syndrome). A harbinger of tumor progression or relapse. Cancer 1992;70(4):877–81.

119. Lossos A, Siegal T. Numb chin syndrome in cancer patients: etiology, response to treatment, and prognostic significance. Neurology 1992;42(6): 1181–4.

120. Horton J, Means ED, Cunningham TJ and Olson KB. The numb chin in breast cancer. J Neurol Neurosurg Psychiatry 1973;36(2):211–6.

121. Lesnick JA, Zallen RD. Numb chin syndrome secondary to metastatic breast disease. J Colo Dent Assoc 1999;78(1):11–4.

122. Myall RW, Morton TH and Worthington P. Melanoma metastatic to the mandible. Report of a case. Int J Oral Surg 1983;12(1):56–9.

123. Halachmi S, Madeb R, Madjar S, Wald M, River Y and Nativ O. Numb chin syndrome as the presenting symptom of metastatic prostate carcinoma. Urology 2000;55(2):286.

124. Aung TH, Po YC and Wong WK. Hepatocellular carcinoma with metastasis to the skull base, pituitary gland, sphenoid sinus, and cavernous sinus. Hong Kong Med J 2002;8(1):48–51.

125. Kistler M, Pribram HW. Metastatic disease of the sella turcica. Am J Roentgenol Radium Ther Nucl Med 1975;123(1):13–21.

126. Komninos J, Vlassopoulou V and Protopapa D, et al. Tumors metastatic to the pituitary gland: case report and literature review. J Clin Endocrinol Metab 2004;89(2):574–80.

127. McCormick PC, Post KD, Kandji AD and Hays AP. Metastatic carcinoma to the pituitary gland. Br J Neurosurg 1989;3(1):71–9.

128. Branch CL,Jr, Laws ER,Jr. Metastatic tumors of the sella turcica masquerading as primary pituitary tumors. J Clin Endocrinol Metab 1987;65(3):469–74.

129. Morita A, Meyer FB and Laws ER,Jr. Symptomatic pituitary metastases. J Neurosurg 1998;89(1):69–73.

130. Schubiger O, Haller D. Metastases to the pituitary–hypothalamic axis. An MR study of 7 symptomatic patients. Neuroradiology 1992;34(2):131–4.

131. Harzallah L, Migaw H, Harzallah F and Kraiem C. Diabetes insipidus and panhypopituitarism revealing pituitary metastasis of small cell lung carcinoma: a case report. Ann Endocrinol (Paris) 2005;66(2 Pt 1):117–20.

132. Ginsberg LE. Neoplastic diseases affecting the central skull base: CT and MR imaging. AJR Am J Roentgenol 1992;159(3):581–9.

133. Glenn LW. Innovations in neuroimaging of skull base pathology. Otolaryngol Clin North Am 2005;38(4):613–29.

134. Durden DD, Williams DW,3rd. Radiology of skull base neoplasms. Otolaryngol Clin North Am 2001;34(6):1043,64, vii.

135. Franca C, Levin-Plotnik D, Sehgal V, Chen GT and Ramsey RG. Use of three-dimensional spiral computed tomography imaging for staging and surgical planning of head and neck cancer. J Digit Imaging 2000;13(2 Suppl 1):24–32.

136. Post MJ, Mendez DR, Kline LB, Acker JD and Glaser JS. Metastatic disease to the cavernous sinus: clinical syndrome and CT diagnosis. J Comput Assist Tomogr 1985;9(1):115–20.

137. Yoshizumi K, Korogi Y and Sugahara T, et al. Skull base tumors: evaluation with contrast-enhanced MP-RAGE sequence. Comput Med Imaging Graph 2001;25(1):23–31.

138. Ishida H, Mohri M and Amatsu M. Invasion of the skull base by carcinomas: histopathologically evidenced findings with CT and MRI. Eur Arch Otorhinolaryngol 2002;259(10):535–9.

139. Brillman J, Valeriano J and Adatepe MH. The diagnosis of skull base metastases by radionuclide bone scan. Cancer 1987;59(11):1887–91.

140. Fukumoto M, Osaki Y and Yoshida D, et al. Dual-isotope SPECT diagnosis of a skull base metastasis causing isolated unilateral hypoglossal nerve palsy. Ann Nucl Med 1998;12(4):213–6.

141. Fukui MB, Blodgett TM and Meltzer CC. PET/CT imaging in recurrent head and neck cancer. Semin Ultrasound CT MR 2003;24(3):157–63.

142. Ganly I, Patel SG and Singh B, et al. Complications of craniofacial resection for malignant tumors of the skull base: report of an International Collaborative Study. Head Neck 2005;27(6):445–51.

143. Ganly I, Patel SG and Singh B, et al. Craniofacial resection for malignant melanoma of the skull base: report of an international collaborative study. Arch Otolaryngol Head Neck Surg 2006;132(1):73–8.
144. Patel SG, Singh B and Polluri A, et al. Craniofacial surgery for malignant skull base tumors: report of an international collaborative study. Cancer 2003;98(6):1179–87.
145. Carrillo JF, Rivas Leon B, Celis MA, Ponce-de-Leon S and Ochoa-Carrillo FJ. Anterolateral and lateral skull base approaches for treatment of neoplastic diseases. Am J Otolaryngol 2004;25(1):58–67.
146. Jia G, Zhang J and Wu Z. Diagnosis and treatment of skull base metastasis. Zhonghua Yi Xue Za Zhi 1998;78(10):761–2.
147. Hanbali F., DeMonte F. Metastatic tumors of the skull base. In: Sawaya R, eds. Intracranial Metastases: Current Management Strategies. Elmsford, NY: Blackwell/Futura, 2004.
148. Vikram B, Chu FC. Radiation therapy for metastases to the base of the skull. Radiology 1979;130(2):465–8.
149. Ampil FL. Palliative radiation therapy for metastases in base of skull and cranial nerves. Acta Oncol 1988;27(3):293–4.
150. Ransom DT, Dinapoli RP and Richardson RL. Cranial nerve lesions due to base of the skull metastases in prostate carcinoma. Cancer 1990;65(3):586–9.
151. Francel PC, Bhattacharjee S and Tompkins P. Skull base approaches and gamma knife radiosurgery for multimodality treatment of skull base tumors. J Neurosurg 2002;97(5 Suppl):674–6.
152. Miller RC, Foote RL and Coffey RJ, et al. The role of stereotactic radiosurgery in the treatment of malignant skull base tumors. Int J Radiat Oncol Biol Phys 1997;39(5):977–81.
153. Cmelak AJ, Cox RS, Adler JR, Fee WE,Jr and Goffinet DR. Radiosurgery for skull base malignancies and nasopharyngeal carcinoma. Int J Radiat Oncol Biol Phys 1997;37(5):997–1003.
154. Iwai Y, Yamanaka K. Gamma Knife radiosurgery for skull base metastasis and invasion. Stereotact Funct Neurosurg 1999;72 Suppl 1:81–7.
155. Iwai Y, Yamanaka K and Yoshimura M. Gamma knife radiosurgery for cavernous sinus metastases and invasion. Surg Neurol 2005;64(5):406,10; discussion 410.
156. Kocher M, Voges J, Staar S, Treuer H, Sturm V and Mueller RP. Linear accelerator radiosurgery for recurrent malignant tumors of the skull base. Am J Clin Oncol 1998;21(1):18–22.
157. Seymore CH, Peeples WJ. Cranial nerve involvement with carcinoma of prostate. Urology 1988;31(3):211–3.
158. Hall SM, Buzdar AU and Blumenschein GR. Cranial nerve palsies in metastatic breast cancer due to osseous metastasis without intracranial involvement. Cancer 1983;52(1):180–4.

8. Pediatric Brain Metastasis from Extraneural Malignancies: A Review

Stewart Goldman, MD, María E. Echevarría, MD, Jason Fangusaro, MD

Introduction

Brain metastasis is a well described and common complication in adult patients with cancer. It is estimated that between 25–40% of all adults with malignancies will develop brain metastasis [1–4]. This is particularly common in patients with melanoma, lung cancer, breast cancer and gastrointestinal tract neoplasms [5, 6]. In pediatric patients with solid tumors, however, the incidence of brain metastases is exceedingly rare. Most of the recent literature suggests that the overall incidence of brain metastases in pediatric oncology patients ranges from 1–10% [1–4]. The specific risk, however, is not yet well defined and seems dependent upon unique patient and tumor characteristics. Since the spectrum of tumors in pediatrics greatly differs from adult malignancies, it is difficult to extrapolate the adult experience to pediatrics. In this chapter, we will attempt to better define the presence of brain metastases in pediatric oncology. We will describe the most common patient symptoms, presentations and risk factors, and we will review the pediatric malignancies at highest risk for this rare event. Finally, we will focus upon current evaluation, treatment and outcomes in pediatric patients with brain metastases.

One of the major challenges in understanding brain metastases is agreeing upon a common and accepted definition. There are basically two major modes of spread to the brain from extracranial solid tumors. A malignancy can spread to the brain when it arises from adjacent structures that invade the meninges and brain parenchyma. This phenomenon often can be observed with osteosarcoma and rhabdomyosarcoma, tumors that can occur in parameningeal locations with higher risk of developing local tumor invasion [7, 8]. Typically, this type of spread leads to extradural metastasis. Hematogenous spread from distant locations is another major mechanism of metastasis to the brain. Invariably, hematogenous spread leads to intradural/intraparenchymal disease, and most researchers agree that these patients, indeed, have true brain metastases. Some of the literature, however, excludes patients who develop brain involvement from adjacent spread, and therefore, it is difficult to compare studies and estimate an overall incidence. Also, some studies include patients who develop solitary leptomeningeal spread of disease while others exclude these patients unless they have a distinct intracranial tumor component in addition to leptomeningeal disease. Another confounding variable is agreeing upon what specific malignancies to include when evaluating brain metastases in pediatrics. Many researchers focus upon one particular tumor type in evaluating brain metastases and often specific tumors may be excluded from a series. For the purposes of this review, we will discuss studies that both include and exclude CNS disease from adjacent spread and leptomeningeal dissemination, and we will evaluate the most common types of pediatric malignancies to develop brain metastases.

Among the numerous types of pediatric tumors, the most common tumors that develop brain metastases include: acute lymphoblastic leukemia, acute myelogenous leukemia, non-Hodgkin's lymphoma, Ewing's sarcoma, neuroblastoma, Wilm's tumor and other kidney tumors, soft tissue sarcomas including rhabdomyosarcoma, osteosarcoma, melanoma, hepatoblastoma, retinoblastoma and germ cell tumors. There are rare case reports on other much less common tumor types, including myxofibrosarcoma of the heart, nasopharyngeal carcinoma, pleural pulmonary blastoma and adrenal cortical carcinoma, but the majority of pediatric patients with brain metastases develop spread from one of the aforementioned malignancies [9–12].

Interestingly, the presentation and symptoms of the patients with solid tumor metastases does not seem to vary considerably among different tumor types. Leukemias and lymphomas, however, may present with some unique caveats and characteristics, and for this reason, they will be considered separately from the solid tumors.

Solid Tumors

Symptoms and Presentation

The symptoms experienced by patients with brain metastases from most solid tumors seem most often related to increased intracranial pressure. Parasuraman et al found that among 21 patients who developed brain metastases from rhabdomyosarcoma and Ewing's sarcoma, all 21 showed signs of elevated intracranial pressure, focal neurologic deficits, seizures or altered sensorium. In this series, each patient developed symptoms before imaging was obtained [13]. Similarly, Paulino et al found that among 30 patients with brain metastases from a variety of solid tumors, the most common signs and symptoms were emesis, headache, seizures, hemiparesis, extremity weakness, loss of balance and incoordination [14]. Other large series have found very similar presenting symptoms including loss of consciousness, nystagmus, ptosis, head tilt, speech difficulties and impaired vision

[15]. Since it is rare for most pediatric tumors to spread to the brain and spinal cord, routine surveillance imaging is often not obtained. Typically, one or more symptoms lead to detailed imaging revealing a CNS lesion. Rarely, a new brain lesion may be found on imaging done because of widely metastatic disease evaluations or because of a specific tumor's tendency to spread to the CNS. For example, clear cell sarcoma of the kidney has a tendency to spread to the brain, and routine brain imaging is often obtained [16].

Another common finding among many patients who develop brain metastases is the presence of metastasis to other distant sites. Kebudi et al found that among 16 pediatric patients who eventually developed brain metastases, 12 of 16 presented initially with some type of distant metastasis including lung, bone, bone marrow, abdomen and liver disease. Three of 16 patients presented with brain metastasis at initial diagnosis, but all three of these patients had metastatic disease elsewhere, including the lung and abdomen. CNS disease was never an isolated finding in any of the 16 patients [15]. On the whole, it appears that brain metastases are seen in the setting of recurrent or multiply recurrent disease that already has metastasized elsewhere throughout the body [1]. One theory is that as we become better at treating pediatric malignancies with multi-modal therapies, we are prolonging survival in a group of patients with aggressive disease who previously would have had much shorter life spans. Brain metastasis may be part of the natural history of these diseases that was previously unseen with early patient death [1,17–20]. This change in metastatic spread has become most evident in many of the solid tumors which will be evaluated separately below.

Ewing's Sarcoma

Ewing's sarcoma represents a family of tumors that include Ewing's sarcoma of bone, extraosseous Ewing's sarcoma and peripheral neuroectodermal tumor (PNET) of bone and soft tissue. It the second most common bone tumor in pediatrics with approximately 200–250 new cases each year in patients less than 20 years of age [21–23]. The most common locations for Ewing's sarcoma to develop are the pelvis, the femur and the ribs. Therapy consists of surgery, chemotherapy and radiation therapy depending upon extent of disease at diagnosis [21, 23]. Advances in chemotherapy have improved survival to 70% in localized disease while the outcome for patients with metastatic disease is much less promising [22]. Ewing's sarcoma has a tendency to metastasize to the lung, bone and bone marrow, but brain metastases have been documented throughout the literature [13, 15, 24].

Parasuraman et al. reported the experience at St. Jude Children's Research Hospital. Eleven of 335 Ewing's sarcoma (3.3%) patients developed brain metastases. Slightly more than half of these brain lesions appeared to develop from hematogenous spread while the remainder appeared to develop from direct extension of adjacent lesions [13]. Bouffet et al. evaluated a variety of solid tumors and found that 3 of 54 (5.4%) Ewing's sarcoma patients developed brain metastases, making it the most common solid tumor in their study to develop metastatic brain lesions. This group excluded lesions thought to develop from direct extension, so this 5.4% of Ewing's patients represents a group thought to develop brain metastases solely from hematogenous or lymphatic spread [1]. A recent survey by Kebudi et al. evaluated 1100 pediatric patients with solid tumors over a 13 year period. They found that 4 of 84 (4.8%) patients with Ewing's sarcoma developed metastatic brain lesions [15]. Other series have shown that between 3–16% of Ewing's sarcoma patients will eventually develop brain metastases, making it one of the most common extra-cranial solid tumors to develop brain metastases cited in the literature [1–3,14,25,26].

Major risk factors identified that lead to the development of brain metastases in Ewing's sarcoma patients are the presence of relapsed/progressive disease and metastases to other distant locations, particularly to lungs. Most series show that the patients who develop brain metastases from Ewing's sarcoma are those with recurrent disease that has already spread to other distant sites [14, 25]. The large retrospective study at St. Jude Research Hospital revealed that the majority of patients with brain metastases from Ewing's sarcoma either had some type of metastatic disease at diagnosis or recurrence. There were, however, 4 patients with Ewing's sarcoma in which the brain was either the sole or initial site of relapsed disease [13]. These patients present with symptoms suggestive of increased intracranial pressure. Most patients with brain metastases from Ewing's sarcoma are identified after the presentation of new neurologic symptoms that lead to further evaluation. Brain and spinal surveillance imaging are not routinely obtained in most cases.

Treatment for patients with Ewing's sarcoma that has spread to the CNS consists of surgical resection, usually for symptomatic or single lesions. Whole brain radiotherapy and chemotherapy are also utilized, but outcomes are typically dismal with few long-term survivors beyond a year from detection of CNS lesions [27–29].

Osteosarcoma

Osteosarcoma is a pediatric malignancy of bone often seen in adolescence. It is the most common type of primary bone tumor seen in pediatrics. Primary lesions are most often seen in the femur, proximal tibia, and pelvis, however, it can be seen in a variety of bones throughout the body including the bones adjacent to the CNS [30]. Multimodal therapy consisting of surgery and chemotherapy successfully treats approximately 60–70% of patients [31]. Those patients with metastatic disease at diagnosis continue to have dismal outcomes despite aggressive surgery and chemotherapy [30]. Typically, the lungs have been the dominant site of metastasis and relapse, but spread to the brain has been well reported [1, 7, 15, 32].

A retrospective review conducted at St. Jude Research Hospital described 254 patients treated for osteosarcoma over a 27 year period. Sixteen of 254 (6.3%) developed metastatic brain lesions, and only 3 of these were felt secondary to direct extension/invasion of lesions adjacent to the CNS [7]. A series from M.D. Anderson reported their experience with 87 consecutive osteosarcoma patients treated over a twenty-six year period.They found 13% incidence of brain metastases[17]. The few series reported in the literature documenting brain metastases in pediatric osteosarcoma reveal an incidence ranging from 4 to 13%, again making osteosarcoma one of the more common pediatric solid tumors to develop brain lesions [1–3,14,17,25,26].

There are very few specific risk factors that have been identified in the osteosarcoma population that lead to an increased risk of brain metastasis. Again, a pattern is seen similar to other solid tumors whereas those patients with multiply recurrent disease and widely metastatic disease to other distant locations such as the lungs have the highest risk of developing spread to the brain [7, 32]. Sometimes, if the osteosarcoma is in a bone adjacent to the CNS, more thorough brain imaging may be undertaken, but in general, the brain metastatic lesions are identified after the development of new symptoms suggestive of increased intracranial pressure. The treatment strategies employed in these patients are similar to those for numerous types of sarcomas that have spread to the CNS. Surgical resection is undertaken when possible, usually for symptomatic or isolated lesions, followed by radiotherapy with or without chemotherapy depending upon previous exposure and the patient's organ function [28, 29, 33]. Although outcomes are dismal, there have been some cases of prolonged survival utilizing multimodal therapies and prolonged chemotherapy [7, 32].

Rhabdomyosarcoma

Rhabdomyosarcoma is a member of a group of tumors known as the soft tissue sarcomas which are thought to develop from primitive mesenchyme. The soft tissue sarcomas arise from primitive muscle, connective, supportive and vascular tissue. In general, these tumors have a high rate of recurrence, metastasize via the blood stream and/or lymphatics and are more common in adults than in children. Rhabdomyosarcoma is the most common soft tissue sarcoma of childhood and represents about 50% of all childhood sarcomas. It accounts for about 10% of all childhood solid tumors and 6% of pediatric malignancies. There are approximately 250 new cases each year in the United States [34, 35]. Clinical outcome is dependent upon tumor site, group and staging. Treatments consisting of surgery, chemotherapy and radiation therapy have resulted in close to 70% overall survival at 5 years [35]. Metastases develop in up to 20% of cases, and the most common metastatic sites include the lungs, lymph nodes, and bone marrow [34].Brain metastases have been documented throughout the literature both by local invasion of adjacent tumors and hematogenous spread [1,8,13–15].

Parasuraman et al. found that over a 36 year period, there were 419 patients diagnosed and treated for rhabdomyosarcoma at St. Jude Children's Research Hospital. On retrospective analysis, 10 of 419 (2.4%) had CNS involvement. Only one patient who had a parameningeal primary tumor had brain involvement at diagnosis. All other patients developed metastatic brain disease upon recurrence or further progression. The brain was the first site of relapse in 3 patients.

Six patients developed brain metastases after the development of disease at other distant sites including the lung, bones, lymph nodes and other soft tissue sites [13]. Interestingly, rhabdomyosarcoma patients developed spread to the brain significantly earlier than Ewing's sarcoma patients evaluated during the same time period. Rhabdomyosarcoma patients developed brain metastases at a median of 12 months from initial diagnosis compared to 22 months in Ewing's patients [13].

In another large retrospective analysis, Paulino and colleagues. found that among 104 patients with rhabdomyosarcoma evaluated at University of Iowa Hospitals and Clinics over a 35 year period, 7 of 104 (6.7%) developed brain metastases. All seven patients had concurrent or prior history of hematogenous spread to other distant sites at the time the metastatic brain disease was discovered [14]. Other large series that have included the evaluation of rhabdomyosarcoma have found similar risk ranging from 5–10% [1, 15, 17, 24].

The presenting symptoms experienced by these patients are very similar to those symptoms as seen in most other patients with solid tumors that have spread to the CNS.It again appears that those patients with recurrent disease and distant metastases to other locations are at highest risk for developing brain metastases [1, 8, 14, 15]. Interestingly, the group of patients with parameningeal rhabdomyosarcoma may be at greater risk for intracranial extension. Parameningeal rhabdomyosarcoma can develop in many sites including the mastoid, nasopharynx, paranasal sinuses, parapharyngeal space, pterygopalatine fossa and infratentorial fossa [8]. Risk factors associated with meningeal spread are the presence of cranial nerve palsies, skull base erosion and obvious intracranial tumor extension [8, 36, 37]. Historically, these patients have been treated more aggressively because of their increased risk of spread to the brain and high risk of recurrent disease.

The treatment strategy in rhabdomyosarcoma involving the CNS is similar to other sarcomas that have spread to the brain. Patients with isolated or symptomatic brain lesions may undergo a surgical resection often followed by a combination of chemotherapy and radiotherapy [13, 28, 29]. Although the outcomes for parameningeal disease has appeared to improve over time with multi-modal therapies, those patients with true CNS spread usually succumb to their disease [8, 13, 29].

Retinoblastoma

Retinoblastoma is the most common primary eye malignancy in children under 15 years of age. It is most often seen during infancy, but it can be seen in older children, and rarely, young adults. It can present sporadically in the first two years of life often with unilateral disease or may present secondary to a genetic mutation in the Rb gene. The genetic variant is typically seen during infancy and commonly presents with bilateral disease. The two major presenting signs of retinoblastoma are leukocoria and strabismus [38, 39]. Current treatment strategies include a combination of surgical removal of the eye known as enucleation, cryotherapy and chemotherapy [40]. This strategy has resulted in very good long term survivals, particularly in patients with localized unilateral disease [41, 42]. Retinoblastoma can metastasize to regional lymph nodes, bone marrow, distant bones and the CNS [43–46]. In a study evaluating 18 consecutive retinoblastoma patients with metastatic disease, 9 out of 18 had CNS disease. Five of the 9 also had evidence of concurrent metastases to other distant sites including bones and bone marrow [45]. Numerous studies have documented that optic nerve involvement in retinoblastoma is one of the most important risk factors for CNS metastasis [47–49]. The lesions associated with metastatic retinoblastoma are usually multiple and occur during the first two years of initial treatment [50].

A distinct recognized phenomenon is the so called trilateral retinoblastoma (TRb) in which a patient with hereditary retinoblastoma develops a tumor within the pineal, suprasellar and/or parasellar region [51]. These lesions often appear several months to years after initial presentation of retinoblastoma and most often occur in children under 4 years of age [52, 53]. Trilateral retinoblastoma has a high mortality rate despite aggressive treatment with chemotherapy, radiation therapy, gamma knife therapy and high dose chemotherapy with autologous hematopoietic cell rescue (Au HCR) [54]. Longer survival has been correlated with earlier tumor diagnosis in asymptomatic patients.

In retinoblastoma, metastatic disease involving brain or other sites and trilateral retinoblastoma require an aggressive combined therapeutic approach. Many patients have been pre-treated with chemotherapy and craniospinal radiation when CNS disease is detected. In extraneural metastatic disease, treatment may result in greater than 50% 5-year survivals in patients that received chemotherapy utilizing ifosfamide, carboplatin and eloposide (ICE) or high-dose chemotherapy with Au HCR [45, 55, 56]. CNS involvement generally carries a poor prognosis and overall survival rates are close to 0% despite aggressive treatment [43–45,57]. There is some preliminary data to suggest that those children with retinoblastoma treated with chemotherapy may have a decreased incidence of trilateral retinoblastoma [58, 59].

Hepatoblastoma

Hepatoblastoma is the most common liver cancer in childhood, accounting for approximately 80% of hepatic tumors. It has been associated with Beckwith-Wiedemann syndrome, Familial Adenomatous Polyposis syndrome, Li-Fraumeni syndrome and Triosmy 18. Clinical presentations include a right upper quadrant mass, abdominal pain, anorexia, anemia and thrombocytosis with a concurrent increase in alpha feto protein (AFP) levels seen in 90% of cases. Surgery is the mainstay of therapy for hepatoblastomas, and the use of pre-operative cisplatin-based chemotherapy has increased the event-free survival up to 80% for tumors completely resected.

The most common site for metastases is the lung, but metastases to bone and brain have been rarely reported. Seven cases have been described in the literature.

Two Patients had metastatic disease at initial diagnosis and 5 palients developed lesions 6 to 32 months after diagnosis. All patients had evidence of lung metastases concurrently or preceding the diagnosis of intracranial involvement [60–65].

Treatment approaches for CNS metastatic disease vary. If an isolated metastatic brain lesion is identified, surgical resection has been advocated followed by local field radiation. For patients with multi-focal disease, whole brain radiation has been utilized as a treatment strategy [60, 61, 65]. Robertson et al. describes the only reported child with prolonged survival. This patient had an isolated brain metastasis with numerous recurrences that was treated with multiple surgical resections, local radiation and chemotherapy [65].

Neuroblastoma

Neuroblastoma (NB) is the most common extra-cranial solid tumor in children, accounting for 8% to 10% of all childhood cancers. In the United States there are about 800 newly diagnosed cases per year with a slight male predominance. The etiology of neuroblastoma is unknown, but a subset of patients exhibits a genetic predisposition to develop this disease (short arm chromosome 16p12–13). Age, stage, and unique molecular defects encountered in tumor cells are important prognostic factors and are used for risk-stratification and treatment assignment. Several factors have been associated with poor outcomes, including N-MYC oncogene amplification, near diploid cell DNA content, an unbalanced gain of chromosome 17q and high expression of TrkB and its ligand.

The management of neuroblastoma includes surgery, chemotherapy, high dose chemotherapy with Au HCR and focal involved field radiotherapy. Specific treatment strategies are determined by a thorough evaluation of tumor stage, patient age, tumor pathology and tumor biology. Infants younger than 1 year have an excellent prognosis, even in the presence of metastatic disease. Older patients with metastatic disease, however, fair poorly, even when treated with aggressive therapy. Less than half of older patients with metastatic disease are cured, even with the use of high-dose therapy followed by Au HCR.

Many children older than 1 year present with extensive or metastatic disease at the time of diagnosis. Metastatic extension can occur via lymphatic and hematogenous Spread. Hematogenous spread occurs most frequently to bone marrow, bone, liver and skin. Rarely, neuroblastoma may spread to lung and brain parenchyma. In neuroblastoma, CNS metastases usually arise from adjacent bone metastasis and true parenchymal brain metastases are rare. Brain metastases may have associated spinal cord metastases [1–3,26,66]. Although dissemination within the central nervous system is rarely seen at diagnosis, the incidence of brain metastasis in children who experience a recurrence varies. Prior to 1980, most cases of brain metastasis were seen in patients with advanced stage neuroblastoma and widespread systemic and cranial disease. Among the largest series reported, the incidence of CNS disease ranges from 1% to 8% [1, 14, 67, 68]. Improving therapies and the subsequent prolongation of survival rates have raised the concern that, analogous to childhood leukemia, the CNS may emerge as a sanctuary for neuroblastoma and become a leading site of recurrent disease. Kramer et al. conducted a retrospective study analyzing all patients with metastatic neuroblastoma who were treated on four consecutive protocols (N4 to N7) at Memorial Sloan-Kettering Cancer Center from 1980 to 1999; 4.4 % (11 out of 251) experienced progressive disease involving the CNS. None had CNS neuroblastoma at the time of diagnosis, but seven patients had bone or bone marrow involvement at diagnosis. These recurrences occurred 5–32 months (median, 12.2 months) from the initial diagnosis. In seven cases, the CNS was the sole site of recurrence. For the newly diagnosed subset, the incidence rate of CNS neuroblastoma increased from 1.7% (N4, N5) to 11.7% (N6, N7) over the years, probably due to more effective curative therapies and, most recently, the use of immunotherapy agents that do not cross the blood brain barrier [69]. No consistent or effective treatment approach exists for patients with neuroblastoma that has spread to the brain. Treatment approaches have included surgical resection, irradiation and/or high dose chemotherapy with Au HCR. Unfortunately these approaches are generally ineffective and the majority of patients with CNS neuroblastoma die from their disease.

Germ Cell Tumors

Extracranial germ cell tumors account for approximately 3–5% of all pediatric malignancies in patients less than 20 years old. These tumors consist of a variety of tumors with differing histologies. The most common locations include the ovaries, testis, coccyx, mediastinum and, rarely, other midline structures [70, 71]. Approximately 15–30% of patients develop some type of distant metastasis, including spread to regional lymph nodes, lungs, liver or bones. Treatment consisting of surgical resection/biopsy followed by chemotherapy leads to greater than 80% overall survival [70]. Brain metastases from germ cell tumors have been well documented in the adult population and can be seen in approximately 1–2% of adults upon diagnosis [72]. Spread to the brain is less well characterized in pediatrics, though it has been documented [15, 73].

The largest retrospective study exclusively evaluating brain metastases in pediatric germ cell tumors was conducted at St. Jude Research Hospital over a 40 year period. During this period, the authors identified 16 of 206 (7.8%) patients with germ cell tumors with spread to the CNS. Among these 16 patients, 2 were diagnosed with brain metastasis at diagnosis, 12 developed CNS disease later during their disease course, and finally, 2 patients were found to have CNS disease at autopsy evaluation. Fourteen of 16 patients had concurrent pulmonary metastasis at the time brain disease was identified. The authors noted that as modern therapy changed during their study period, there was a decreased incidence of brain metastases in this population, suggesting the effectiveness of improved therapies [73]. Kebudi also documented spread of germ cell tumors to the CNS. Among 1100 children with a variety of solid tumors evaluated over a thirteen year period, 16 patients had brain metastases. Among these 16 patients, 2 patients had primary germ cell tumors. One patient had a choriocarcinoma and the other had an endodermal sinus tumor. Both of these patients died from disease progression/complications [15].

Spunt et al. noted that those patients at highest risk for developing brain metastasis were those with extragonadal tumors, high stage disease at presentation and those with choriocarcinoma as a component of the primary tumor. Most patients had symptoms suggestive of increased intracranial pressure including nausea, emesis, headaches, and seizures. Only a small number of patients survived, and the majority of patients died of progressive disease despite a variety of therapies, including surgical resection, further chemotherapy, and radiation therapy [73].

Melanoma

Malignant melanoma in children is extremely rare, accounting for 1% of all pediatric malignancies [74–77]. The clinical course appears to be similar to that in adults, and prognosis is dependent on stage [74,76–79]. In adults, brain metastases are often multifocal and can develop in approximately 20–30% of patients. Brain metastases account for approximately 50% of deaths in these patients [80–82]. The risk of developing CNS lesions in patients with evidence of visceral metastases has been estimated to be 40 to 70% [80]. Patients with multiple brain metastases have an 80% incidence of systemic disease [83, 84]. Intra-lesional hemorrhage is one characteristic feature of these lesions. 20% of adult patients experience a catastrophic event secondary to intracranial bleeding within the tumor [82, 85, 86]. Overall survival depends upon the ability of multiple modalities to control systemic disease.

In the pediatric population the incidence of brain metastases in patients with melanoma has been reported between 8% and 18% [76, 77, 87]. In a large retrospective series over a 33 year period, 8 out of 44 melanoma patients (18%) developed brain metastases during the course of the disease, at a median of 20 months from diagnosis (range 0–50 months). In accordance with the adult literature, the majority of these CNS metastases had multiple lesions, and five of these patients had evidence of concurrent metastases and/or developed metastases at other distant sites (lungs, lymph nodes, bone, skin and bowel). One patient had a single brain metastasis as the initial presentation. Although 63% of these patients had evidence of intratumoral bleeding, these episodes were usually clinically insignificant. All patients received corticosteroids and whole brain radiation. One underwent surgical resection of a solitary lesion, and three received adjuvant chemotherapy. Finally, one patient received chemotherapy and immunotherapy with interferon-alpha-2a. Five of the eight patients died from their CNS metastatic lesions at a median of 5 months (range 2–10 months) after diagnosis of CNS involvement [87].

Immediate treatment for CNS metastatic malignant melanoma is corticosteroids. Chemotherapy plays a limited role and the palliative effect of radiation therapy is short lived [88–91]. Surgical resection is appropriate, especially for solitary lesions. In adults, surgery followed by whole brain radiation has resulted in a median of 8–14 month survival [83, 84, 90, 92]. The use of adjuvant interferon-alpha-2a has recently been associated with better overall survival rates in patients with localized melanomas, suggesting the agent has anti-tumor activity [93]. In children, brain metastases usually represent a terminal disease stage, but Rodriguez-Galindo et al. reports a single long-term survivor without evidence of disease at 34 months follow up. This patient had a single brain metastasis as the first manifestation of the disease and was treated with total surgical resection, followed by whole brain radiation, adjuvant chemotherapy and interferon-alpha-2a [87].

Renal Tumors

Renal tumors represent approximately 6 % of childhood malignancies and usually present with the development of an asymptomatic abdominal mass, abdominal pain and/or hematuria. Primary renal tumors in children less than 15 years of age include Wilm's tumor, rhabdoid tumors and clear cell sarcoma of the kidney. Renal cell carcinoma and congenital mesoblastic nephroma, though rare, do occur. For the purposes of this review, we will focus on the most common entities.

Wilm's Tumor

Wilm's tumor is the most common primary malignant renal tumor of childhood, accounting for 6–7% of childhood cancer, with an incidence of approximately 500 cases per year in the United States in patients age less than 15 Years old. It appears to be more common among African Americans and least common in the East Asian population. The male to female ratio is 0.92: 1 for those with unilateral disease and 0.6:1 for those with bilateral disease. The median age at diagnosis is approximately 3.5 years [94].

Wilm's tumor is well recognized as part of several congenital malformation syndromes such as: WAGR syndrome (Wilm's tumor, aniridia, genitourinary malformations and mental retardation), Denys-Drash (triad of congenital nephropathy, Wilms tumor and intersex disorders) and Beckwith-Wiedemann syndrome (congenital exomphalos, macroglossia, and gigantism). It has been also associated, to a lesser extent, with neurofibromatosis, Soto's syndrome (excessive physical growth, mild mental retardation, delayed motor development, delayed cognitive and social development, hypotonia and speech impairments) and has been observed in families affected by Li-Fraumeni syndrome (cancer predisposition syndrome associated with sarcomas, breast cancer, leukemia, melanoma, colon cancer, pancreatic cancer and brain tumors) [94].

Outcome and overall survival rates depend upon many factors such as tumor size, patient's age, histology (favorable vs. anaplastic), and staging, which in the past have been predictive of risk for tumor recurrence or progression. The National

Wilm's Tumor Study Group studies (NWTS) report 4 year overall survival (OS) rates that vary from 95.6% in Stage I favorable histology to 16.7% in Stage IV, with diffuse anaplasia. Treatment is multimodal and includes surgery, chemotherapy and/or radiation, depending on staging and pathology. Recent research has focused on identification of additional prognostic factors, ideally ones that are independent of stage and histology, which could be employed for further stratification of therapy according to the risk of recurrence. These include possible molecular genetic prognostic factors (loss of heterozygosity of chromosome 16q and/or 1p), tumor cell DNA content and tumor level of telomerase expression [94].

Wilm's tumor usually metastasizes to lungs, regional lymph nodes, liver and, rarely to bone or brain. The development of brain metastases has been associated most commonly with prior or concurrent lung metastases [1, 3, 25, 26, 66, 95]. Vannucci et al. found that prior to 1975, Wilm's tumor was the most common cause of brain metastases in autopsies done in patients with solid tumors, accounting for 13% (4 out of 31 patients) of the cases [26]. The majority of the cases with CNS involvement presented initially with advance disease to lung. Since these reports, the introduction of new chemotherapeutic agents and treatment modalities have changed this pattern. The most recent series showed that the overall incidence of brain metastases in Wilm's tumor is among 0.6% to 4.7% [61]. Two single institutional reviews done at the Centre Léon Bérard (France) and at the University of Iowa Hospitals and Clinics (USA) reported that 1.3% and 1% of children with Wilm's tumor developed brain metastases respectively [1, 14]. Kebudi et al. reviewed 43 patients diagnosed with Wilm's tumor over an 11 year period in Turkey [15]. Two patients (4.7%) developed brain metastases, both with lung metastases at diagnosis. Lowis et al. reviewed the data over a 16-year period from three consecutive United Kingdom Wilm's Tumour Studies (UKW 1, 2, and 3 trials) and found that 7 out of 1249 (0.6%) children developed brain metastases between 2 to 27 months after initial diagnosis [95]. In these 4 series, none of the patients presented with initial CNS metastatic disease, and the majority had lung involvement at diagnosis or developed lung disease prior to the CNS lesions [1, 14, 15, 95].

As compared to the approximately 50% long term survivors in patients with non-CNS metastatic Wilm's tumor [96], the development of brain metastasis has been associated with rapid clinical deterioration. The majority of patients have died despite different treatment approaches including surgical resection of isolated CNS lesions, whole brain irradiation and chemotherapy [1, 14, 15]. Lowis and colleagues, however, have reported on 3 out of 7 survivors with brain metastasis alive for a mean of 63 months after recurrence. They were treated with radiotherapy and chemotherapy including carboplatin, etoposide and ifosfamide [95]. The authors conclude that this group of patients does not necessarily have a poor prognosis, and indeed, in the absence of pulmonary metastasis or resistance to chemotherapy, there remains a chance of cure with multimodal treatments (surgery, chemotherapy and local radiotherapy) [95].

Clear Cell Sarcoma of the Kidney (CCSK)

CCSK is the second most common pediatric renal neoplasm, compromising 3–6% of primary childhood renal tumors [97, 98]. Management is multimodal and includes surgical resection/biopsy, chemotherapy and radiation therapy. Despite aggressive treatment, it is associated with aggressive clinical behavior, and higher rates of relapse and death compared to Wilm's tumor. The most common sites of metastases are bone, regional lymph nodes, lung, liver and brain [16, 99]. Usually, bone metastases precede the development of distant metastatic lesions. Recent reports from the National Wilm's Tumor Study Group and the International Society for Pediatric Oncology (SIOP) have indicated that the brain may have surpassed the bone as the most common site of CCSK metastases, but the reason remains unclear [99, 100].

CCSK is also characterized by an extended period during which metastases may present [94], probably due to improved detection and longer survival. As treatment and survival continue to improve, the incidences can be expected to increase even more [101]. Park et al. suggested that the relapse and metastasis of clear cell sarcoma are probably due to re-growth of micrometastases which are present at early disease stages [16]. In a recent series, Radulescu et al. described the treatment and outcomes of 8 CCSK patients treated in separate institutions in the United States, Canada and the United Kingdom who developed brain metastases over a 3 year period [102]. Two out of eight patients had evidence of metastatic disease at diagnosis (lungs and bone marrow), but none had brain metastases. All patients achieved complete response to initial therapy. The recurrences occurred at a median of 24.5 months after initial diagnosis (range 12–53 months). Patients were treated with surgery, variable courses of chemotherapy (ICE +/− other agents), with or without radiation. Four patients received high –dose chemotherapy with Au HCR. At a median follow-up of 30 months from the time of recurrence, 6 patients. were alive without disease. The authors suggest that ICE chemotherapy, together with radiation therapy and surgery, provided a reasonable salvage treatment regimen for recurrent CCSK that has metastasized to the brain [102]. The role of high dose-chemotherapy remains undefined, despite several encouraging reports [103–105].

Rhabdoid Tumor of the Kidney

Malignant rhabdoid tumor of the kidney (MRTK) is a rare aggressive cancer that occurs more frequently in infants, with approximately 85% of cases diagnosed within the first 2 years of life. It accounts for 1.5% of renal cancers in children enrolled on the National Wilm's Tumor Study (NWTS) Group trials. MRTK has a dismal prognosis and more than 80% of children die within 1 year of diagnosis. Treatment consists of surgical resection, followed by chemotherapy and radiation therapy. Patients less than 1 year of age at diagnosis tend to have the worst outcomes and are more prone to develop CNS tumors, possibly because they are at increased risk of harboring the cancer predisposing germ-line mutations *INI1* [106].

Previous studies have reported that 10 to 15% of patients with MRTK develop CNS lesions, often secondary to synchronous or metachronous metastasis. However, second unique primary tumors such as PNET/medulloblastomas, ependymomas or gliomas have been noted. The recent recognition that CNS atypical teratoid/rhabdoid tumors (AT/RT) have deletions of the *INI1* gene indicates that rhabdoid tumors of the kidney and brain are identical or closely related entities. This observation is not surprising because rhabdoid tumors at both locations possess similar histologic, clinical, and demographic features [94, 107].

A total of 30 out of 142 (21%) patients with MRTK studied on NWTS 1–5 had CNS involvement at some point. Patients ranged in age from 1 to 26 months and 86% were less than 1 year of age at diagnosis. Ten patients had pathologic analysis of CNS lesions, and in 6 cases it was consistent with a second primary brain tumor (4 PNETs, 1 Anaplastic Astrocytoma, 1 AT/RT). All but one infant died despite aggressive treatment. The authors concluded that higher tumor stage and presence of CNS lesions were both factors predictive of a poor survival rate [106]. Treatment for CNS AT/RT consists of surgery, chemotherapy and radiation therapy. Radiation and aggressive chemotherapy appear to improve some patients' outcomes, but most succumb to their disease [108].

Leukemia and Lymphoma

The spread of acute leukemia to the CNS first became clinically evident in the late 1950s throughout the early 1960s. As effective systemic chemotherapy was developed and survival times increased the CNS became the most frequent site of initial relapse/metastasis [109]. As modern leukemia therapies evolved metastasis/spread to the CNS was reported in some series as high as 80–85% [109, 110]. CNS leukemia has been postulated by many to develop as a result of leukemic metastasis. Mastrengelo in 1970 performed cytogenetic analysis of lymphoblasts from patients' marrow and CSF and found their karyotypes to be similar [111]. It is hypothesized that these leukemic cells metastasize through hematogenous spread. Hematogenous spread could occur through venous endothelium or secondary to petechial hemorrhages that occur during times of thrombocytopenia [112]. Choroid plexus, tissue which has a vast network of capillaries has been implicated as a site of leukemic infiltration into the CNS [113, 114]. Alternatively, leukemic metastasis to the CNS may occur through direct extension from cranial bone marrow. Bridging veins between the bone marrow and superficial arachnoid or along the perineum have been hypothesized to be of importance [113–118]. The recognition of metastasis to the CNS has lead to the development of CNS prophylaxis as part of the standard treatment regimens for pediatric leukemia.

Acute Lymphoblastic Leukemia (ALL)

In Acute Lymphoblastic Leukemia (ALL), less than 5% of children present with CNS leukemia at diagnosis [115]. Present therapy stratifies patients by risk factors including the presence or absence of CNS disease at diagnosis, age (<1 years old and >10 years old are considered higher risk), initial WBC count and others as noted in Table 1[114]. CNS leukemia disease status is defined by the leukemia cells in the lumber CSF and/or related neurologic symptoms as depicted in Table 2.

After stratification into risk groups patients are placed onto treatment regimens which modulate the number of induction agents as well as the length of therapy and the use of delayed and double delayed intensification. All of these modern regimens include various intensities of CNS prophylaxis. With current regimens it can be expected that less than 10% of patients will have CNS metastasis, and those "average risk" patients will have less than a 5% chance of developing CNS involvement as part of relapse [116–118].

Patient with leukemic infiltration of the CNS may present with headache, nausea, vomiting, lethargy, nuchal rigidity, irritability and other signs of increased intracranial pressure including papilledema. Cranial nerve involvement may manifest as an isolated event such as numbness in the face or ocular motor palsies. The most common cranial nerves involved are the 7th, 3rd, 4th, and 6th cranial nerves. Cranial nerve involvement has also been reported as presenting with tinnitus and vertigo. In the modern era CNS involvement presenting with spinal cord compression or other mass effect is infrequent. With the advent of central nervous system prophylaxis as part of standard therapy, CNS metastases that occur while on treatment infrequently present with symptoms. It is more likely to be diagnosed with routine cytological examination of the CSF obtained during the administration of intrathecal medications for CNS prophylaxis.

The treatment of metastatic disease to the central nervous system is dependent upon the previous therapy used to prevent CNS disease. Overall, once a CNS metastases has been discovered, further CNS remissions can be obtained in more than 90% of patients. These remissions, however, are frequently of short duration, usually lasting from 1–2 years. Most patients develop recurrent CNS disease or relapses at other sites such as the bone marrow, testes or multiple sites [119–121].

The use of intrathecal medications such as methotrexate will induce CNS remissions in the majority of patients with CNS metastasis, however, unless this is followed by prolonged continuation of intrathecal therapy and or craniospinal irradiation, relapses will occur within 3–4 months time [122–124]. Other treatment approaches such as high dose systemic methotrexate have been shown to induce CNS remissions. New agents such as topotecan, busulfan, mafosfamide and the combinations of methotrexate, ARA-C and hydrocortisone have been used to induce remission [125].

Treatment Regimens for CNS Prophylaxis

The regimens used to prevent CNS metastasis are dependent upon the CNS staging (see Table 1) and the systemic therapy prescribed. Presently, children who present

Table 1. Prognostic Factors in Pediatric ALL

Initial WBC	Age at Diagnosis
Sex	Ploidy
	Hyperdiploidy +
	Hypodiploidy, Pseudodiploidy, Tetraploidy –
	Near Haploidy - -
FAB morphology	Immunologic subtype
Hgb level	Tumor burden—organomegally,
	Lymphadenopathy, mediastinal mass
Platelet count	Rate of remission (marrow M1 day7)

Table 2. Definitions of Central Nervous System disease status at diagnosis based on CSF findings

CNS-1	No Lymphoblasts
CNS-2	<5 WBCs/ul with definite blasts on cytocentrifuge exam
CNS-3	>5 WBC/ul with + lymphoblasts (or CN palsies)

without CNS disease will receive intrathecal chemotherapy (methotrexate, vs. triple intrathecal therapy such as methotrexate, hydrocortisone and ARA-C). Patients with very high risk disease such as, but not limited to extremely high white count, younger age (less than 1 years old), T-cell disease and lymphomatous presentation still may be considered for intrathecal therapy and cranial radiation for CNS prophylaxis[114].

Acute Myelogenous Leukemia (AML)

CNS metastasis in AML presents an important issue not just at diagnosis but throughout treatment. Leukemic spread to the CNS at diagnosis is more prevalent with AML than ALL. Initial CSF cytology is positive in 5–15% of newly diagnosed AML patients [126]. Reports form the US and German cooperative groups have found the highest incidence of AML with CNS involvement to be in the myelomonocytic and monoblastic (FAB M4 andM5) groups [127]. Pui reviewed two consecutive AML trials from St. Jude's Children's research center and found CNS disease at diagnosis correlated with high WBC and age under 2years old at diagnosis [126]. Abbott et al. at St. Jude reviewed the significance of CNS metastasis at diagnosis in 290 consecutive patients with AML treated on four consecutive institutional protocols. He found no difference in Event Free Survival (EFS) for those with or without CNS involvement at diagnosis [128]. CNS prophylaxis is part of the standard of care for pediatric AML therapy. The exclusion of CNS prophylactic therapy has resulted in CNS relapse rates as high as 20% [126, 130].

CNS involvement with AML may manifest as headaches, nausea, vomiting, cranial nerve findings, photophobia were papilledema, or it may present with mass effect from a chloroma.

Lymphoma

Lymphomas (Hodgkin's and on-Hodgkin's disease) constitute approximately 10% of all childhood cancers in developed countries [131]. In series from equatorial Africa, lymphomas (mainly Burkitt's) account for 50% of childhood cancers [132]. The incidence of CNS involvement at diagnosis and relapse is dependent on the histological classification of the lymphoma. In the U.S. data gathered from the surveillance epidemiology end results (SEER) project from 1985–90, revealed 57% of lymphoma cases in kids less than 15 were NHL and the remainder were Hodgkin's The incidence of lymphomas remains much lower in children than adults, with more extra-nodal disease in children compared to adults and a much narrower range of histological appearances.

Non-Hodgkin's Lymphomas

CNS involvement at presentation is rarely seen with lymphoblastic lymphomas. CNS involvement can include meningeal infiltration, cranial nerve involvement and intracerebral or paraspinal disease. However, it is not commonly seen without concurrent bone marrow involvement [133, 134]. Paraspinal involvement in the equatorial Burkitt's lymphoma is frequent. In a review by Magrath in 1991, 15% of African patients with Burkitt's lymphoma presented with paraplegia[132]. Burkitt's lymphoma in the U.S., however, rarely has CNS involvement as compared to those patients affected in Africa [133]; Finally, anaplastic large cell (Ki-1) lymphomas have a greater propensity to have metastatic involvement of the CNS at the time of diagnosis.

Data from national cooperative groups reveal the low incidence of CNS metastasis for Lymphoblastic lymphoma. In two large trials, 7% of patients treated on the cooperative study, NHL-BFM 86, and 8 % of patients on the LMT 81 SFOP study presented with CNS involvement [135, 136]. Modern protocols include intrathecal medications for CNS prophylaxis as well as systemic agents with good CNS penetration, such as high –dose methotrexate. Primary CNS lymphomas in childhood are usually associated with underlying immunodeficiencies and/or acquired immune deficiencies which are beyond the scope of this chapter.

Hodgkin's lymphoma

CNS involvement in Hodgkin's disease is exceedingly rare. Metastasis to the brain from Hodgkin's lymphoma was first reported in an adult in 1967 [137]. Zimmerman's review of patients with CNS metastasis reported only 0.22% of cases involved Hodgkin's disease, and no pediatric patients were reported [138]. Reports of CNS involvement in pediatrics are vanishingly rare.

CNS metastasis in pediatric leukemias and lymphomas carry substantial risk both at diagnosis and as a site of relapse/ progression. Treatment modalities not only include chemotherapeutic agents with good CNS penetration, as but also the use of intrathecal and intra-ommaya chemotherapy. Finally, cranial and/or craniospinal irradiation are utilized as both a prophylactic and therapeutic treatment measure, in a risk adaptive manner.

References

1. Bouffet E, Doumi N, Thiesse P, et al. Brain metastases in children with solid tumors. Cancer 1997;79(2):403–10.
2. Deutsch M, Albo V, Wollman MR. Radiotherapy for cerebral metastases in children. International journal of radiation oncology, biology, physics 1982;8(8):1441–6.
3. Deutsch M, Orlando S, Wollman M. Radiotherapy for metastases to the brain in children. Medical and pediatric oncology 2002;39(1):60–2.
4. Subramanian A, Harris A, Piggott K, Shieff C, Bradford R. Metastasis to and from the central nervous system–the 'relatively protected site'. The lancet oncology 2002;3(8):498–507.
5. Aronson SM, Garcia JH, Aronson BE. Metastatic Neoplasms of the Brain: Their Frequency In Relation to Age. Cancer 1964;17:558–63.
6. Le Chevalier T, Smith FP, Caille P, Constans JP, Rouesse JG. Sites of primary malignancies in patients presenting with cerebral metastases. A review of 120 cases. Cancer 1985;56(4):880–2.
7. Marina NM, Pratt CB, Shema SJ, Brooks T, Rao B, Meyer WH. Brain metastases in osteosarcoma. Report of a long-term survivor and review of the St. Jude Children's Research Hospital experience. Cancer 1993;71(11): 3656–60.
8. Meazza C, Ferrari A, Casanova M, et al. Evolving treatment strategies for parameningeal rhabdomyosarcoma: the experience of the Istituto Nazionale Tumori of Milan. Head & neck 2005;27(1):49–57.
9. Wagner AS, Fleitz JM, Kleinschmidt-Demasters BK. Pediatric adrenal cortical carcinoma: brain metastases and relationship to NF-1, case reports and review of the literature. Journal of neuro-oncology 2005;75(2):127–33.
10. Kim DG, Lee SY, Chung SK, Park SK, Chun YK, Chi JG. Brain metastasis from myxofibrosarcoma of the heart. Acta neurochirurgica 1997;139(1):88–9.
11. Ngan RK, Yiu HH, Cheng HK, Chan JK, Sin VC, Lau WH. Central nervous system metastasis from nasopharyngeal carcinoma: a report of two patients and a review of the literature. Cancer 2002;94(2):398–405.
12. Yusuf U, Dufour D, Jenrette JM, 3rd, Abboud MR, Laver J, Barredo JC. Survival with combined modality therapy after intracerebral recurrence of pleuropulmonary blastoma. Medical and pediatric oncology 1998;30(1):63–6.

13. Parasuraman S, Langston J, Rao BN, et al. Brain metastases in pediatric Ewing sarcoma and rhabdomyosarcoma: the St. Jude Children's Research Hospital experience. J Pediatr Hematol Oncol 1999;21(5):370–7.

14. Paulino AC, Nguyen TX, Barker JL, Jr. Brain metastasis in children with sarcoma, neuroblastoma, and Wilms' tumor. International journal of radiation oncology, biology, physics 2003;57(1):177–83.

15. Kebudi R, Ayan I, Gorgun O, Agaoglu FY, Vural S, Darendeliler E. Brain metastasis in pediatric extracranial solid tumors: survey and literature review. Journal of neuro-oncology 2005;71(1):43–8.

16. Park DY, Kim YM, Chi JG. Intracranial metastasis from clear cell sarcoma of the kidney–a case report. Journal of Korean medical science 1997;12(5): 473–6.

17. Baram TZ, van Tassel P, Jaffe NA. Brain metastases in osteosarcoma: incidence, clinical and neuroradiological findings and management options. Journal of neuro-oncology 1988;6(1):47–52.

18. Danziger J, Wallace S, Handel SF, deSantos LA. Metastatic osteogenic sarcoma to the brain. Cancer 1979;43(2):707–10.

19. Espana P, Chang P, Wiernik PH. Increased incidence of brain metastases in sarcoma patients. Cancer 1980;45(2):377–80.

20. Gercovich FG, Luna MA, Gottlieb JA. Increased incidence of cerebral metastases in sarcoma patients with prolonged survival from chemotherapy. Report of cases of leiomysarcoma and chondrosarcoma. Cancer 1975;36(5):1843–51.

21. Bernstein M, Kovar H, Paulussen M, et al. Ewing's sarcoma family of tumors: current management. The oncologist 2006;11(5):503–19.

22. Marec-Berard P, Philip T. Ewing sarcoma: the pediatrician's point of view. Pediatr Blood Cancer 2004;42(5):477–80.

23. Thacker MM, Temple HT, Scully SP. Current treatment for Ewing's sarcoma. Expert review of anticancer therapy 2005;5(2):319–31.

24. Sarno JB, Wiener L, Waxman M, Kwee J. Sarcoma metastatic to the central nervous system parenchyma: a review of the literature. Medical and pediatric oncology 1985;13(5):280–92.

25. Graus F, Walker RW, Allen JC. Brain metastases in children. The Journal of pediatrics 1983;103(4):558–61.

26. Vannucci RC, Baten M. Cerebral metastatic disease in childhood. Neurology 1974;24(10):981–5.

27. Bindal RK, Sawaya RE, Leavens ME, Taylor SH, Guinee VF. Sarcoma metastatic to the brain: results of surgical treatment. Neurosurgery 1994;35(2):185–90; discussion 90–1.

28. Ogose A, Morita T, Hotta T, et al. Brain metastases in musculoskeletal sarcomas. Japanese journal of clinical oncology 1999;29(5):245–7.

29. Postovsky S, Ash S, Ramu IN, et al. Central nervous system involvement in children with sarcoma. Oncology 2003;65(2):118–24.

30. Longhi A, Errani C, De Paolis M, Mercuri M, Bacci G. Primary bone osteosarcoma in the pediatric age: state of the art. Cancer treatment reviews 2006;32(6):423–36.
31. Hayden JB, Hoang BH. Osteosarcoma: basic science and clinical implications. The Orthopedic clinics of North America 2006;37(1):1–7.
32. Wexler LH, DeLaney TF, Saris S, Horowitz ME. Long-term survival after central nervous system relapse in a patient with osteosarcoma. Cancer 1993;72(4):1203–8.
33. Salvati M, Cervoni L, Caruso R, Gagliardi FM, Delfini R. Sarcoma metastatic to the brain: a series of 15 cases. Surgical neurology 1998;49(4):441–4.
34. Rodeberg D, Arndt C, Breneman J, et al. Characteristics and outcomes of rhabdomyosarcoma patients with isolated lung metastases from IRS-IV. Journal of pediatric surgery 2005;40(1):256–62.
35. Rodeberg D, Paidas C. Childhood rhabdomyosarcoma. Seminars in pediatric surgery 2006;15(1):57–62.
36. Gasparini M, Lombardi F, Gianni C, Lovati C, Fossati-Bellani F. Childhood rhabdomyosarcoma with meningeal extension: results of combined therapy including central nervous system prophylaxis. American journal of clinical oncology 1983;6(4):393–8.
37. Raney RB, Meza J, Anderson JR, et al. Treatment of children and adolescents with localized parameningeal sarcoma: experience of the Intergroup Rhabdomyosarcoma Study Group protocols IRS-II through -IV, 1978–1997. Medical and pediatric oncology 2002;38(1):22–32.
38. Balmer A, Zografos L, Munier F. Diagnosis and current management of retinoblastoma. Oncogene 2006;25(38):5341–9.
39. Abramson DH, Beaverson K, Sangani P, et al. Screening for retinoblastoma: presenting signs as prognosticators of patient and ocular survival. Pediatrics 2003;112(6 Pt 1):1248–55.
40. Shields CL, Shields JA, De Potter P. New treatment modalities for retinoblastoma. Current opinion in ophthalmology 1996;7(3):20–6.
41. Kaneko A, Suzuki S. Eye-preservation treatment of retinoblastoma with vitreous seeding. Japanese journal of clinical oncology 2003;33(12): 601–7.
42. Suzuki S, Kaneko A. Management of intraocular retinoblastoma and ocular prognosis. International journal of clinical oncology / Japan Society of Clinical Oncology 2004;9(1):1–6.
43. Antoneli CB, Ribeiro KC, Steinhorst F, Novaes PE, Chojniak MM, Malogolowkin M. Treatment of retinoblastoma patients with chemoreduction plus local therapy: experience of the AC Camargo Hospital, Brazil. J Pediatr Hematol Oncol 2006;28(6):342–5.
44. Antoneli CB, Steinhorst F, de Cassia Braga Ribeiro K, et al. Extraocular retinoblastoma: a 13-year experience. Cancer 2003;98(6):1292–8.

45. Gunduz K, Muftuoglu O, Gunalp I, Unal E, Tacyildiz N. Metastatic retinoblastoma clinical features, treatment, and prognosis. Ophthalmology 2006;113(9):1558–66.
46. Namouni F, Doz F, Tanguy ML, et al. High-dose chemotherapy with carboplatin, etoposide and cyclophosphamide followed by a haematopoietic stem cell rescue in patients with high-risk retinoblastoma: a SFOP and SFGM study. Eur J Cancer 1997;33(14):2368–75.
47. Khelfaoui F, Validire P, Auperin A, et al. Histopathologic risk factors in retinoblastoma: a retrospective study of 172 patients treated in a single institution. Cancer 1996;77(6):1206–13.
48. Shields CL, Shields JA, Baez K, Cater JR, De Potter P. Optic nerve invasion of retinoblastoma. Metastatic potential and clinical risk factors. Cancer 1994;73(3):692–8.
49. Shields CL, Shields JA, Baez KA, Cater J, De Potter PV. Choroidal invasion of retinoblastoma: metastatic potential and clinical risk factors. The British journal of ophthalmology 1993;77(9):544–8.
50. Hurwitz RL. Principles & Practice of Pediatric Oncology. 5th Edition ed. Philadelphia: Lippincott Williams & Wilkins; 2006.
51. Singh AD, Shields CL, Shields JA. New insights into trilateral retinoblastoma. Cancer 1999;86(1):3–5.
52. Kivela T. Trilateral retinoblastoma: a meta-analysis of hereditary retinoblastoma associated with primary ectopic intracranial retinoblastoma. J Clin Oncol 1999;17(6):1829–37.
53. De Potter P. Current treatment of retinoblastoma. Current opinion in ophthalmology 2002;13(5):331–6.
54. Paulino AC. Trilateral retinoblastoma: is the location of the intracranial tumor important? Cancer 1999;86(1):135–41.
55. Rodriguez-Galindo C, Wilson MW, Haik BG, et al. Treatment of metastatic retinoblastoma. Ophthalmology 2003;110(6):1237–40.
56. Rodriguez-Galindo C, Wilson MW, Haik BG, et al. Treatment of intraocular retinoblastoma with vincristine and carboplatin. J Clin Oncol 2003;21(10):2019–25.
57. Zelter M, Damel A, Gonzalez G, Schwartz L. A prospective study on the treatment of retinoblastoma in 72 patients. Cancer 1991;68(8):1685–90.
58. Meadows AT, Shields CL. Regarding chemoreduction for retinoblastoma and intracranial neoplasms. Archives of ophthalmology 2004;122(10):1570–1; author reply 1.
59. Shields CL, Shields JA, Meadows AT. Chemoreduction for retinoblastoma may prevent trilateral retinoblastoma. J Clin Oncol 2000;18(1):236–7.
60. Begemann M, Trippett TM, Lis E, Antunes NL. Brain metastases in hepatoblastoma. Pediatric neurology 2004;30(4):295–7.
61. Curless RG, Toledano SR, Ragheb J, Cleveland WW, Falcone S. Hematogenous brain metastasis in children. Pediatric neurology 2002;26(3):219–21.

62. Endo EG, Walton DS, Albert DM. Neonatal hepatoblastoma metastatic to the choroid and iris. Archives of ophthalmology 1996;114(6):757–61.

63. Feusner JH, Krailo MD, Haas JE, Campbell JR, Lloyd DA, Ablin AR. Treatment of pulmonary metastases of initial stage I hepatoblastoma in childhood. Report from the Childrens Cancer Group. Cancer 1993;71(3): 859–64.

64. Nagle SB, Deolekar MV, Dhamnaskar P. Hepatoblastoma with complete regeneration of liver and with metastasis to lungs and brain within six months after partial hepatectomy–a case report. Indian journal of pathology & microbiology 1996;39(2):147–9.

65. Robertson PL, Muraszko KM, Axtell RA. Hepatoblastoma metastatic to brain: prolonged survival after multiple surgical resections of a solitary brain lesion. J Pediatr Hematol Oncol 1997;19(2):168–71.

66. Allen JC. Brain Metastases. Boston: Kluwer Academic Publishers; 1990.

67. Kellie SJ, Hayes FA, Bowman L, et al. Primary extracranial neuroblastoma with central nervous system metastases characterization by clinicopathologic findings and neuroimaging. Cancer 1991;68(9):1999–2006.

68. Shaw PJ, Eden T. Neuroblastoma with intracranial involvement: an ENSG Study. Medical and pediatric oncology 1992;20(2):149–55.

69. Kramer K, Kushner B, Heller G, Cheung NK. Neuroblastoma metastatic to the central nervous system. The Memorial Sloan-kettering Cancer Center Experience and A Literature Review. Cancer 2001;91(8):1510–9.

70. Gobel U, Calaminus G, Schneider DT, Schmidt P, Haas RJ. Management of germ cell tumors in children: approaches to cure. Onkologie 2002;25(1): 14–22.

71. Rescorla FJ, Breitfeld PP. Pediatric germ cell tumors. Current problems in cancer 1999;23(6):257–303.

72. Bokemeyer C, Nowak P, Haupt A, et al. Treatment of brain metastases in patients with testicular cancer. J Clin Oncol 1997;15(4):1449–54.

73. Spunt SL, Walsh MF, Krasin MJ, et al. Brain metastases of malignant germ cell tumors in children and adolescents. Cancer 2004;101(3):620–6.

74. Davidoff AM, Cirrincione C, Seigler HF. Malignant melanoma in children. Ann Surg Oncol 1994;1(4):278–82.

75. Miller RW, Young JL, Jr., Novakovic B. Childhood cancer. Cancer 1995;75 (1 Suppl):395–405.

76. Pratt CB, Palmer MK, Thatcher N, Crowther D. Malignant melanoma in children and adolescents. Cancer 1981;47(2):392–7.

77. Tate PS, Ronan SG, Feucht KA, Eng AM, Das Gupta TK. Melanoma in childhood and adolescence: clinical and pathological features of 48 cases. Journal of pediatric surgery 1993;28(2):217–22.

78. Bader JL, Li FP, Olmstead PM, Strickman NA, Green DM. Childhood malignant melanoma. Incidence and etiology. The American journal of pediatric hematology/oncology 1985;7(4):341–5.
79. Rao BN, Hayes FA, Pratt CB, et al. Malignant melanoma in children: its management and prognosis. Journal of pediatric surgery 1990;25(2):198–203.
80. Amer MH, Al-Sarraf M, Baker LH, Vaitkevicius VK. Malignant melanoma and central nervous system metastases: incidence, diagnosis, treatment and survival. Cancer 1978;42(2):660–8.
81. Budman DR, Camacho E, Wittes RE. The current causes of death in patients with malignant melanoma. Eur J Cancer 1978;14(4):327–30.
82. Retsas S, Gershuny AR. Central nervous system involvement in malignant melanoma. Cancer 1988;61(9):1926–34.
83. Hagen NA, Cirrincione C, Thaler HT, DeAngelis LM. The role of radiation therapy following resection of single brain metastasis from melanoma. Neurology 1990;40(1):158–60.
84. Stevens G, Firth I, Coates A. Cerebral metastases from malignant melanoma. Radiother Oncol 1992;23(3):185–91.
85. Enzmann DR, Kramer R, Norman D, Pollock J. Malignant melanoma metastatic to the central nervous system. Radiology 1978;127(1):177–80.
86. Somaza S, Kondziolka D, Lunsford LD, Kirkwood JM, Flickinger JC. Stereotactic radiosurgery for cerebral metastatic melanoma. Journal of neurosurgery 1993;79(5):661–6.
87. Rodriguez-Galindo C, Pappo AS, Kaste SC, et al. Brain metastases in children with melanoma. Cancer 1997;79(12):2440–5.
88. Carella RJ, Gelber R, Hendrickson F, Berry HC, Cooper JS. Value of radiation therapy in the management of patients with cerebral metastases from malignant melanoma: Radiation Therapy Oncology Group Brain Metastases Study I and II. Cancer 1980;45(4):679–83.
89. Fletcher WS, Daniels DS, Sondak VK, et al. Evaluation of cisplatin and DTIC in inoperable stage III and IV melanoma. A Southwest Oncology Group study. American journal of clinical oncology 1993;16(4):359–62.
90. Katz HR. The relative effectiveness of radiation therapy, corticosteroids, and surgery in the management of melanoma metastatic to the central nervous system. International journal of radiation oncology, biology, physics 1981;7(7):897–906.
91. Merimsky O, Inbar M, Gerard B, Chaitchik S. Fotemustine–an advance in the treatment of metastatic malignant melanoma. Melanoma research 1992;2 (5–6):401–6.
92. Choi KN, Withers HR, Rotman M. Metastatic melanoma in brain. Rapid treatment or large dose fractions. Cancer 1985;56(1):10–5.
93. Kirkwood JM, Strawderman MH, Ernstoff MS, Smith TJ, Borden EC, Blum RH. Interferon alfa-2b adjuvant therapy of high-risk resected cutaneous

melanoma: the Eastern Cooperative Oncology Group Trial EST 1684. J Clin Oncol 1996;14(1):7–17.

94. Dome JS. Principles & Practice of Pediatric Oncology. 5th Edition ed. Philadelphia: Lippincott Williams & Wilkins; 2006.

95. Lowis SP, Foot A, Gerrard MP, et al. Central nervous system metastasis in Wilms' tumor: a review of three consecutive United Kingdom trials. Cancer 1998;83(9):2023–9.

96. Groot-Loonen JJ, Pinkerton CR, Morris-Jones PH, Pritchard J. How curable is relapsed Wilms' tumour? The United Kingdom Children's Cancer Study Group. Archives of disease in childhood 1990;65(9):968–70.

97. Beckwith JB. Wilms' tumor and other renal tumors of childhood: a selective review from the National Wilms' Tumor Study Pathology Center. Human pathology 1983;14(6):481–92.

98. Argani P, Perlman EJ, Breslow NE, et al. Clear cell sarcoma of the kidney: a review of 351 cases from the National Wilms Tumor Study Group Pathology Center. The American journal of surgical pathology 2000;24(1):4–18.

99. Seibel NL SJ, Anderson JR. Outcome of clear cell sarcoma of the kidney (CCSK) treated on the National Wilms Tumor Study-5 (NWTS). Proc Am Soc Clin Oncol 2006;24:502S.

100. Furtwangler R RH, Beier R. Clear-cell sarcoma (CCSK) of the kidney-results of the SIOP 93–01/GPOH trial. Pediatric Blood and Cancer 2005;45:423.

101. Sahjpaul RL, Ramsay DA, de Veber LL, Del Maestro RF. Brain metastasis from clear cell sarcoma of the kidney–a case report and review of the literature. Journal of neuro-oncology 1993;16(3):221–6.

102. Radulescu VC, Gerrard M, Moertel C, et al. Treatment of recurrent clear cell sarcoma of the kidney with brain metastasis. Pediatr Blood Cancer 2007.

103. Hempel L, Sauerbrey A, Zintl F, Weirich A, Lemmer A, Graf N. Successful management of a child with clear cell sarcoma of the kidney (CCSK) and multifocal bone metastases at diagnosis. Medical and pediatric oncology 2003;41(1):97–9.

104. Pein F, Michon J, Valteau-Couanet D, et al. High-dose melphalan, etoposide, and carboplatin followed by autologous stem-cell rescue in pediatric high-risk recurrent Wilms' tumor: a French Society of Pediatric Oncology study. J Clin Oncol 1998;16(10):3295–301.

105. Yumura-Yagi K, Inoue M, Wakabayashi R, et al. Successful double autografts for patients with relapsed clear cell sarcoma of the kidney. Bone marrow transplantation 1998;22(4):381–3.

106. Tomlinson GE, Breslow NE, Dome J, et al. Rhabdoid tumor of the kidney in the National Wilms' Tumor Study: age at diagnosis as a prognostic factor. J Clin Oncol 2005;23(30):7641–5.

107. Walker DaP, G and Punt, J and Taylor, R. Brain and Spinal Tumors of Childhood: Arnold Publishing; 2004.

108. Zimmerman MA, Goumnerova LC, Proctor M, et al. Continuous remission of newly diagnosed and relapsed central nervous system atypical teratoid/rhabdoid tumor. Journal of neuro-oncology 2005;72(1):77–84.

109. Evans AE, Gilbert ES, Zandstra R. The increasing incidence of central nervous system leukemia in children. (Children's Cancer Study Group A). Cancer 1970;26(2):404–9.

110. Hardisty RM, Norman PM. Meningeal leukaemia. Archives of disease in childhood 1967;42(224):441–7.

111. Mastrangelo R, Zuelzer WW, Ecklund PS, Thompson RI. Chromosomes in the spinal fluid: evidence for metastatic origin of meningeal leukemia. Blood 1970;35(2):227–35.

112. West RJ, Graham-Pole J, Hardisty RM, Pike MC. Factors in pathogenesis of central-nervous-system leukaemia. British medical journal 1972;3(5822): 311–4.

113. de Queiroz AC, Ribeiro DA. [Brain changes in leukemias. Histopathological aspects of choroid plexus involvement]. Arquivos de neuro-psiquiatria 1978;36(4):332–9.

114. Margolin JF PD. Principals and Practice of Pediatric Oncology. 3rd ed. Philadelphia: Lippincott-Raven; 1997.

115. Bleyer WA. Central nervous system leukemia. Pediatric clinics of North America 1988;35(4):789–814.

116. Gelber RD, Sallan SE, Cohen HJ, et al. Central nervous system treatment in childhood acute lymphoblastic leukemia. Long-term follow-up of patients diagnosed between 1973 and 1985. Cancer 1993;72(1):261–70.

117. Pullen J, Boyett J, Shuster J, et al. Extended triple intrathecal chemotherapy trial for prevention of CNS relapse in good-risk and poor-risk patients with B-progenitor acute lymphoblastic leukemia: a Pediatric Oncology Group study. J Clin Oncol 1993;11(5):839–49.

118. Tubergen DG, Gilchrist GS, O'Brien RT, et al. Prevention of CNS disease in intermediate-risk acute lymphoblastic leukemia: comparison of cranial radiation and intrathecal methotrexate and the importance of systemic therapy: a Childrens Cancer Group report. J Clin Oncol 1993;11(3):520–6.

119. Bast RJ SS, Reynolds C. Autologous Bone Transplantation. Houston: M.D. Anderson Hospital and Tumor Institute; 3–6.

120. Bleyer WA, Poplack DG. Prophylaxis and treatment of leukemia in the central nervous system and other sanctuaries. Seminars in oncology 1985;12(2): 131–48.

121. George SL, Ochs JJ, Mauer AM, Simone JV. The importance of an isolated central nervous system relapse in children with acute lymphoblastic leukemia. J Clin Oncol 1985;3(6):776–81.

122. Duttera MJ, Bleyer WA, Pomeroy TC, Leventhal CM, Leventhal BG. Irradiation, methotrexate toxicity, and the treatment of meningeal leukaemia. Lancet 1973;2(7831):703–7.

123. Sullivan MP, Vietti TJ, Fernbach DJ, Griffith KM, Haddy TB, Watkins WL. Clinical investigations in the treatment of meningeal leukemia: radiation therapy regimens vs. conventional intrathecal methotrexate. Blood 1969;34(3): 301–19.
124. Sullivan MP, Vietti TJ, Haggard ME, Donaldson MH, Krall JM, Gehan EA. Remission maintenance therapy for meningeal leukemia: intrathecal methotrexate vs. intravenous bis-nitrosourea. Blood 1971;38(6):680–8.
125. Balis F SJ. Remission induction of meningeal leukemia with high dose intravenous methotrexate. Proc Am Soc Clin Oncol 1984;202(3).
126. Pui CH, Dahl GV, Kalwinsky DK, et al. Central nervous system leukemia in children with acute nonlymphoblastic leukemia. Blood 1985;66(5):1062–7.
127. Grier HE, Gelber RD, Camitta BM, et al. Prognostic factors in childhood acute myelogenous leukemia. J Clin Oncol 1987;5(7):1026–32.
128. Abbott BL, Rubnitz JE, Tong X, et al. Clinical significance of central nervous system involvement at diagnosis of pediatric acute myeloid leukemia: a single institution's experience. Leukemia 2003;17(11):2090–6.
129. Dahl GV, Simone JV, Hustu HO, Mason C. Preventive central nervous system irradiation in children with acute nonlymphocytic leukemia. Cancer 1978;42(5):2187–92.
130. Lampkin BC, Masterson M, Sambrano JE, Heckel JL, Jones G. Current chemotherapeutic treatment strategies in childhood acute nonlymphocytic leukemia. Seminars in oncology 1987;14(4):397–406.
131. Ries LA MR. Cancer in Children. National Institute of Health Publication 1994.
132. Magrath IT. African Burkitt's lymphoma. History, biology, clinical features, and treatment. The American journal of pediatric hematology/oncology 1991;13(2):222–46.
133. Haddy TB, Adde MA, Magrath IT. CNS involvement in small noncleaved-cell lymphoma: is CNS disease per se a poor prognostic sign? J Clin Oncol 1991;9(11):1973–82.
134. Sariban E, Edwards B, Janus C, Magrath I. Central nervous system involvement in American Burkitt's lymphoma. J Clin Oncol 1983;1(11): 677–81.
135. Meadows AT, Sposto R, Jenkin RD, et al. Similar efficacy of 6 and 18 months of therapy with four drugs (COMP) for localized non-Hodgkin's lymphoma of children: a report from the Childrens Cancer Study Group. J Clin Oncol 1989;7(1):92–9.
136. Shad A MI. Principals and Practice of Pediatric Oncology. 3rd ed. Philadelphia: Lippincott-Raven; 1997.
137. Gaelen LH, Levitan S. Solitary intracranial metastasis by Hodgkin's disease. Archives of internal medicine 1967;120(6):740–5.
138. Zimmerman HM. Malignant lymphomas of the nervous system. Acta neuropathologica 1975;Suppl 6:69–74.

9. Brain Metastases in Hematologic Malignancies

Nancy D. Doolittle, Ph.D.

Central nervous system (CNS) involvement in patients with hematologic malignancies is a challenging clinical problem which carries a poor prognosis [1–5]. Hematopoietic and lymphoid neoplasms involve the CNS with varying frequencies. For example, long term disease control in childhood acute lymphoblastic leukemia (ALL) was rare before the recognition of occult CNS disease at diagnosis [6, 7]. Patient outcomes and cure rates dramatically improved once adequate prophylaxis against CNS disease was instituted in the 1970's, as part of standard treatment for childhood ALL [6–8]. Similarly in adult acute lymphoid leukemia, the CNS is a common sanctuary for leukemic cells. The incidence of CNS disease is less than 10% at the time of diagnosis, however increases to 50% to 75% after one year in the absence of CNS prophylaxis [9, 10].

Several investigators have suggested that as new intensive treatment regimens improve the control of systemic cancers including hematologic malignancies, with more patients attaining remission and improved survival, CNS involvement will increase [7, 8, 11, 12]. It is possible that new treatment agents may adequately control systemic disease however may not affect the CNS as a potential sanctuary or reservoir, perhaps due to poor penetration of the blood-brain barrier, thus allowing CNS relapse from disease remission [8, 13–15].

Leis et al. reported CNS relapse in 5 of 24 patients (20.8%) with chronic myeloid leukemia lymphoid blast crisis, Philadelphia chromosome positive acute lymphoblastic leukemia or chronic myeloid leukemia with biphenotypic markers, who were treated on imatinib mesylate protocols [16]. CNS relapse occurred despite peripheral blood (5/5 cases) and bone marrow (3/5 cases) complete responses (CRs). Pharmacokinetic analysis of the patients' plasma and cerebrospinal fluid (CSF) imatinib mesylate levels revealed that imatinib mesylate may not penetrate the CNS at adequate levels to treat occult CNS leukemia [16]. Similar presentations in individual patients have been published as case reports [17, 18]. The blood-brain barrier may prevent adequate penetration of the CNS by systemically administered antileukemic drugs, possibly creating a CNS sanctuary [8,14–16]. CNS failure represents a significant risk factor for this population with advanced disease.

Though intracranial involvement is rare, granulocytic sarcomas may occur in the meninges or in the brain parenchyma [19–21]. The majority of these tumors, which are lesions composed of immature granulocytes, were previously known as "chloromas" because of their typical greenish appearance [19, 20]. Granulocytic sarcomas are usually associated with acute myelogenous leukemia, although they may arise in patients with myeloproliferative or myelodysplastic syndromes [22]. Of interest are recent single case reports of isolated intracerebral granulocytic sarcoma in patients with ALL [20, 21]. This occurrence may again emphasize the importance of the CNS as a sanctuary site, especially in the era of effective control of systemic disease.

During the last 40 years, the classification of lymphoid and myeloid neoplasms has undergone much discussion and reappraisal. Classification systems have been refined secondary to insights gained from immunologic and molecular techniques, as well as clinical advances in the diagnosis and treatment of lymphoma and leukemia [23]. In 1994, the International Lymphoma Study Group (ILSG) published the revised European-American Classification of Lymphoid Neoplasms (the REAL classification) [24]. The World Health Organization later adopted the approach of the REAL classification for lymphoid malignancies, applied the same principles to tumors of other hematopoietic lineages, and published an internationally accepted classification scheme [25].

Central Nervous System Involvement in non-Hodgkin's Lymphoma

This chapter focuses on CNS involvement in non-Hodgkin's lymphoma. During the past 30 years, important progress has been made in understanding non-Hodgkin's lymphoma pathogenesis, as well as in the treatment of this disease. Accompanying this progress has been an improvement in survival rates [5]. Because patients with non-Hodgkin's lymphoma are surviving longer, there is increased risk of developing metastases to the CNS [5].

The CHOP chemotherapy regimen (cyclophosphamide, doxorubicin, vincristine and prednisone) has been the mainstay of treatment for diffuse large B-cell lymphoma (DLBCL) for several decades [26]. The recent addition of the monoclonal antibody rituximab to CHOP chemotherapy (R-CHOP) for the treatment of elderly patients with newly diagnosed DLBCL has led to improved outcomes including an improvement in the cure rate [27–29]. It has been suggested that rituximab may poorly penetrate the blood-brain barrier [30, 31]. Rubinstein et al. reported CSF rituximab concentrations of at most 0.1 % that of matched serum, after intravenous administration of rituximab [32]. With the adoption of R-CHOP as the new standard of care for DLBCL, and with the associated improvement in survival, it is possible that CNS involvement may be seen with increased frequency in the clinical setting.

Patients with previously diagnosed non-Hodgkin's lymphoma may develop clinical evidence of brain or spinal involvement. The most common setting for CNS involvement is during systemic progression of lymphoma; however CNS involvement may herald a relapse [2]. The overall incidence of CNS relapse in patients with non-Hodgkin's lymphoma is reported to be approximately 5% [1, 2, 4] though some series report rates as low as 1% in low-grade lymphomas to a cumulative risk of relapse at 4 years of 39%, in high risk patient groups [4,33–39]. CNS involvement in patients with non-Hodgkin's lymphoma is often rapidly fatal. Most studies report a median survival of 2 to 6 months [6, 33,40–42].

Risk Factors for CNS Metastases

Numerous investigators have attempted to identify patients with non-Hodgkin's lymphoma who are at high risk of developing CNS relapse. The most common risk factor for CNS involvement is histologic subtype [1, 2, 43]. Patients with lymphoblastic lymphoma and Burkitt's lymphoma are at high risk of CNS involvement [2, 4, 34, 35, 43]. Additional risk factors for CNS relapse are: young age [33, 35,43–45], elevated lactate dehydrogenase (LDH) [1, 31, 35, 46], involvement of more than one extranodal site [1, 11, 35, 46], disease stage [1, 31, 33, 40, 43], presence of B symptoms [1, 43], bone marrow involvement [1, 11, 35, 43], low albumin (less than 3.5 g) [35], and involvement of retroperitoneal lymph nodes [35]. The more factors that are present, the higher the risk of CNS relapse [35].

Possible Mechanisms for CNS Metastases

Metastatic invasion of the CNS may involve intracranial structures, the spinal cord, the leptomeninges, or peripheral nerves [8, 47]. Lymphomas may disseminate in several ways: by direct extension into lymphatic channels, direct invasion of the blood vessels thus metastasizing via veins or arteries, or by multicentric neoplastic transformation [47, 48]. The CNS has no lymphatics, so direct extension to the brain and spinal cord by the lymphatic system is not possible. However, lymph nodes in the neck, axilla, mediastinum and retroperitoneal areas when invaded by tumor, may compress adjacent peripheral and cranial nerves and invade the CNS along the involved nerves [47]. Spread to the spinal canal is usually from paravertebral lymph nodes with tumor extending through the intervertebral foramen to produce an epidural mass. Lymphoma may also spread along nerve roots, blood vessels and perineural lymphatics to enter the subarachnoid space, which is in direct continuity with the perivascular Virchow-Robin space [49].

Tumor enters the intracranial cavity by direct extension from lesions in the nasopharynx and cervical lymph nodes along the cranial nerves and meningeal vessels, producing epidural or subdural deposits at the skull base. Most neurologic symptoms are caused by compression of neuronal structures. Hematogeneous spread may sometimes be a factor, however the rarity of solitary intraparenchymal metastases suggests that spread by vascular dissemination is uncommon [47]. Once tumor has reached the CNS, particularly the leptomeninges, it may spread along the spinal fluid pathways to widely involve the nervous system.

CNS Prophylaxis

The absolute role of CNS prophylaxis in patients with non-Hodgkin's lymphoma remains to be determined [2, 5, 50]. The identification of patients who have no CNS involvement at the time of initial non-Hodgkin's lymphoma diagnosis but who have risk factors for CNS relapse at a later point in the disease course is very important [2]. It has been recommended that patients diagnosed with DLBCL, peripheral T-cell non-Hodgkin's lymphoma, and mantle cell lymphoma, with high LDH level, more than one extranodal site, or high risk according to the International Prognostic Index (IPI) classification, should receive CNS prophylaxis with intrathecal or high-dose systemic chemotherapy [4]. Although CNS prophylactic regimens have included systemic and intrathecal drug [2, 35, 42], the optimal CNS prophylactic treatment regimen has not been established [2, 4].

Tomita et al. reported a reduction in the incidence of CNS relapse and an increase in the 5-year overall survival rate after CR in 68 patients with aggressive non-Hodgkin's lymphoma. In their retrospective analysis of 68 patients, 29 received CNS prophylaxis consisting of four doses of intrathecal methotrexate (10 mg/m^2) and hydrocortisone (15 mg/m^2). The other 39 patients did not receive CNS prophylaxis. None of the patients who received CNS prophylaxis recurred in the CNS, whereas 6 patients who did not receive prophylaxis developed CNS recurrence [51]. Haioun et al. reported on 1371 patients with non-Hodgkin's lymphoma treated prospectively with high-dose intravenous methotrexate combined with intrathecal methotrexate or cytarabine [42]. Hollender et al. reported 2514 non-Hodgkin's lymphoma patients without CNS involvement at initial diagnosis, and identified risk factors to guide clinicians in determining which patients should receive CNS prophylaxis [35]. According to these models, patients with high-grade non-Hodgkin's lymphoma should receive intensive intrathecal chemotherapy as well as intravenous chemotherapy, based on disease histology and the presence of five specific risk factors [35].

None-the-less, there is conflicting data in the literature which may be a reason for the wide variation in the use of CNS prophylactic regimens [2, 33, 50]. No data is currently available from prospective controlled clinical trials to definitively guide specific CNS prophylactic measures [5].

Diagnosis of CNS Metastases

Clinical presentation. The most common form of CNS involvement in non-Hodgkin's lymphoma is leptomeningeal metastases with a reported frequency of 4% to 15% [2, 5, 34, 51,53–55]. Leptomeningeal metastases involve the nervous system at multiple levels, thus clinical symptoms cannot easily be localized to a single neuro-anatomic site [2]. Clinically, leptomeningeal involvement often manifests as multifocal neurologic symptoms including cranial nerve involvement, spinal cord symptoms, or headache.

Multiple cranial nerve neuropathies are often noted including diplopia, facial weakness, hearing loss, facial numbness or weakness, and dysphagia [5, 56]. Spinal cord and spinal nerve root involvement often manifests in sensory or motor symptoms [2]. Involvement of nerve roots may cause pain, weakness and sensory loss at the effected spinal level. Patients may experience increased difficulty walking, and neurologic examination may show upper motor neuron involvement with spastic legs, weakness, and increased deep tendon reflexes [2]. Spinal cord involvement may manifest in bladder and bowel dysfunction, especially with involvement of the conus medullaris. Headache is a common symptom of leptomeningeal metastases, and may be caused by increased intracranial pressure secondary to obstruction of CSF flow by the metastases. Increased intracranial pressure may cause nausea, vomiting and mental status changes. Even in the absence of increased intracranial pressure headache may occur.

CNS relapse may involve the brain parenchyma. In contrast to leptomeningeal involvement, metastases to the brain parenchyma is relatively uncommon in non-Hodgkin's lymphoma, with a reported frequency of 1% to 2% [5, 40, 52]. In recent years, with routine use of magnetic resonance imaging (MRI) and modern neuroimaging techniques, brain parenchyma involvement is recognized more frequently [33, 41]. Bokstein et al. reported a series of patients with CNS relapse, in which parenchymal disease was the predominant mode of clinical presentation [41]. The clinical manifestations of parenchymal disease depend on the location and number of lesions. Patients may present with cognitive difficulties, motor or sensory deficits, cranial nerve deficits, seizures, headaches or general symptoms of increased intracranial pressure [57, 58].

CNS relapse may involve spinal cord compression from an epidural mass. Approximately 2% to 5% of patients with non-Hodgkin's lymphoma develop this complication [49, 59]. Paravertebral tumor grows through the intervertebral foramen and then expands within the spinal canal causing progressive weakness and sensory symptoms [2]. Importantly, patients often complain of back pain, often with radiating pain to the dermatome of the involved spinal level. The back pain is important to recognize early, as prompt diagnosis is essential [5]. Patients with epidural metastases require urgent imaging and urgent clinical management.

Neuro-radiologic imaging. Patients with suspected CNS involvement (leptomeningeal or parenchymal metastases) require urgent neuro-imaging of the entire cerebrospinal axis [5]. The imaging modality of choice is MRI with gadolinium enhancement. The blood-brain barrier is leaky in areas of leptomeningeal and parenchymal metastases, allowing for contrast penetration and abnormal enhancement of the lesions [2, 15]. Leptomeningeal metastases may appear as linear or nodular enhancement along cortical sulci, or on the surface of the spinal cord. Large bulky metastases may be seen in the cerebral or spinal subarachnoid space. Brain parenchymal metastases may enhance as single or multiple lesions. Axial fluid-attenuated inversion recovery (FLAIR) and T-1 weighted gadolinium enhanced brain sequences, along with sagittal T-1 weighted gadolinium images of the spine are usually adequate [2]. Additional images may be required depending on the patient's clinical presentation. Grier et al. recommend considerating a radionuclide CSF flow study, especially if there is bulky leptomeningeal disease or hydrocephalus on MRI. A CSF flow study will indicate CSF obstruction, a relative contraindication for intrathecal chemotherapy [2, 5].

Cerebrospinal Fluid Analysis. When leptomeningeal metastases is suspected, the diagnostic work-up should include serial lumbar punctures for CSF analysis. Patients often present with clinical symptoms suggestive of leptomeningeal involvement, have compatible neuro-imaging features, but negative CSF analysis [2, 60]. The CSF analysis includes opening pressure, protein and glucose levels, cell count, cytology, and flow cytometry [2, 5]. In non-Hodgkin's lymphoma with leptomeningeal involvement, many of the analyses are often abnormal; however only cytology is 100% specific [2]. The sensitivity of cytology for diagnosing leptomeningeal metastases with the first lumbar puncture is approximately 50%, and the sensitivity increases to 90% with three repeated lumbar punctures [61]. In combination with cytology, flow cytometry may be of much value in improving the detection of malignant cells in the CSF. Hedge et al. reported 51 patients with newly diagnosed aggressive B-cell lymphoma at risk for CNS involvement. Eleven of 51 patients were diagnosed with CSF involvement by flow cytometry, whereas only 1 of the 11 patients had positive cytology by traditional testing methods [2, 11].

Biopsy. Regarding leptomeningeal metastases, leptomeningeal biopsy may be required in rare cases, in order to determine the histopathologic diagnosis [5]. However leptomeningeal biopsy is not feasible in many clinical situations [61]. In cases with metastatic involvement of the brain parenchyma, which is relatively uncommon in non-Hodgkin's lymphoma, biopsy plays a more important role. When single or multiple brain parenchyma lesions are identified on neuro-imaging studies, non-Hodgkin's lymphoma should not be assumed to be the diagnosis without pathologic verification [5]. This is particularly the case in isolated brain parenchyma metastases.

Isolated CNS Metastases

Though rare, CNS relapse in non-Hodgkin's lymphoma can occur as isolated disease. That is, there is no evidence of lymphoma elsewhere in the body at the time of CNS relapse. Investigators have reported the occurrence of isolated CNS relapse in 3 of 276 cases (1.1%) [31], 16 of 974 cases (1.6%) [42], and 9 of 175 cases (5.2%) [40] of non-Hodgkin's lymphoma. Isolated CNS relapse may involve the leptomeninges, the CSF, the brain parenchyma, and possibly the eyes. Patients with isolated CNS relapse tend to fare better than those who have a concomitant CNS and marrow relapse, or those who experience CNS disease after a recurrence at another site [1, 6, 36]. Haioun et al. reported patients with isolated CNS relapse excluding those with CNS disease occurring in the setting of systemic recurrence, considering as others that in isolated CNS relapse the disease may be treatable, whereas in systemic recurrence, CNS involvement may be an expression of end-stage disease [1, 42, 47].

The International Primary CNS Lymphoma Collaborative Group (IPCG) is a multidisciplinary group convened by the International Extranodal Lymphoma Study Group (IELSG) to address clinical and biologic research questions regarding CNS lymphoma [62]. In a retrospective case series recently assembled by the IPCG, 113 cases of isolated brain parenchyma relapse in non-Hodgkin's lymphoma were assembled from 13 investigators in 8 countries [58]. Cases with no evidence of lymphoma elsewhere in the body at the time of brain parenchyma relapse were eligible. All cases had achieved a CR following initial diagnosis and treatment of non-Hodgkin's lymphoma. Cases with evidence of brain, CSF or leptomeningeal involvement at the time of non-Hodgkin's lymphoma diagnosis were not eligible for the case series review. Inclusive years for the review were 1980 to 2004.

In this series of 113 cases of isolated brain parenchyma relapse, 94 cases (83%) had DLBCL. 76 cases (67%) relapsed in the brain parenchyma less than 3 years after non-Hodgkin's lymphoma diagnosis. Median time from non-Hodgkin's lymphoma diagnosis to isolated brain parenchyma relapse was 1.8 years (minimum 3 months; maximum 15.9 years). The most frequent symptoms were mental status changes (43 cases, 38%), gait/balance disturbances (29 cases, 26%), peripheral sensory or motor symptoms (27 cases, 24%), and headache (23 cases, 20%). CNS disease was assessed by brain imaging in all 113 cases, and by biopsy in 54 cases (48%). Cerebrospinal fluid was positive for lymphoma cells in 11 cases (10%), negative for lymphoma cells in 56 cases (50%), and unknown in 46 cases (40%). Median overall survival in this series was 1.6 years (95% CI: 11 months to 2.6 years) [58]. Though this was a retrospective case series review, it is an attempt to characterize patient and disease characteristics as well as clinical outcomes, in isolated brain parenchyma involvement of non-Hodgkin's lymphoma.

Treatment of CNS Metastases

It is important to distinguish between patients whose CNS disease is the initial site of recurrence from those where CNS disease occurs long after systemic recurrence [1]. In the former group, CNS disease may be potentially treatable; in the latter, CNS recurrence is an expression of end-stage disease, and is unlikely to be amenable to therapeutic strategies with curative intent [1]. Treatment decisions are based on the extent of leptomeningeal and brain parenchyma involvement, the status of systemic disease, and the patient's performance status and quality of life [6]. Conventional treatment options for CNS relapse have included corticosteroids, intrathecal or intraventricular chemotherapy, systemic chemotherapy, or radiotherapy. The use of radiotherapy alone with a curative intent requires craniospinal irradiation, which carries the risk of neurotoxicity [36, 38,63–65].

Involved-field radiation to radiographically evident leptomeningeal disease has been used in an effort to provide relief of radicular pain from involvement of spinal nerve roots, or may help to restore CSF circulation in patients with CSF obstruction [1, 2, 5]. However responses to radiation are often transient [1, 55]. Patients may present with epidural metastases causing rapid progressive spinal cord compression. Urgent treatment is radiotherapy to the involved area. Chemotherapy has been successfully used for epidural disease however is usually reserved for patients without significant neurologic compromise [2, 59].

Leptomeningeal metastases are often treated with intrathecal chemotherapy, systemic chemotherapy or both. Repeated intrathecal treatments may be facilitated by placement of an Ommaya reservoir [2]. The most commonly used intrathecal agents are methotrexate and cytarabine [5]. Cytarabine is available as a slow release (liposomal) formulation, which offers the convenience of less frequent administration. Glantz et al. reported on the efficacy of liposomal cytarabine in a randomized study [66]. Side effects associated with intrathecal delivery of slow release cytarabine may include seizures, aseptic meningitis and arachnoiditis. Methotrexate is often administered intrathecally at a dose of 10 to 12 mg, twice a week. Methotrexate also carries the potential for side effects, especially in patients who have received prior cranial radiotherapy for parenchymal or leptomeningeal metastases [2, 63, 67].

Despite various treatments initiated after CNS relapse (intrathecal chemotherapy, intraventricular chemotherapy, systemic chemotherapy, radiotherapy, and various combinations thereof), the median survival is reported to be 2 to 4 months [1, 33, 40, 44]. Bokstein et al. reported the feasibility and response to pre-radiation chemotherapy in 23 patients with CNS relapse [41]. Treatment was high-dose methotrexate (3.5 g/m^2) and intra-CSF cytarabine (50 mg). Radiation treatment was reserved for treatment failures [41]. Systemic methotrexate-based chemotherapy yielded an initial CNS response rate of 100% and a 47% concomitant systemic response. However durable responses were rare and the overall median survival in this series was 6 months. The authors concluded that future trials should evaluate alternative modalities to enhance drug delivery to the CNS [41].

Glantz et al. reported on 16 patients with leptomeningeal metastases from solid tumors, who were treated with high-dose intravenous methotrexate (8 grams/m^2) alone [66]. Prolonged cytotoxic CSF concentrations of methotrexate were achieved with intravenous methotrexate. Overall survival in the intravenous group was 13.8 months, versus 2.3 months in the intrathecal group, which was a significant survival benefit in patients with leptomeningeal metastases [66].

Dose-Intensive Chemotherapy

When treating CNS relapse of non-Hodgkin's lymphoma, several investigators have reported rapid CNS responses from conventional therapies however responses are of short duration and overall survival remains poor [1, 40, 41, 55, 68]. Most of these investigators have discussed the importance of new treatment approaches aimed at both enhancing drug delivery into the CNS and improving dose intensity at sites of systemic disease [1, 6, 41, 55, 68]. Such strategies should yield improved survival compared with conventional-dose chemotherapy alone [69].

Patients who have relapsed non-Hodgkin's lymphoma with and without CNS involvement are often treated with high-dose chemotherapy and autologous hematopoietic stem cell transplantation [2]. Long term survival can be achieved in patients with a history of CNS involvement using this treatment strategy [69, 70]. However, available data shows that CNS disease should be cleared before treatment with transplantation [71–73]. A retrospective examination of 1464 lymphoma patients in the European Bone Marrow Transplant Lymphoma Registry, revealed 62 cases of CNS involvement [71]. Patients who had prior CNS relapse but were cleared of CNS disease at the time of bone marrow transplantation, had a 5-year progression free survival of 42%, whereas patients with CNS involvement at the time of transplantation had a progression free survival of 9% at 71 months, a significant difference from the other group.

van Besien et al. reported on the impact of prior or current CNS disease on the outcome of high-dose chemotherapy in hematologic malignancies [72]. Twenty patients who had prior CNS involvement but no active disease at the time of transplant, showed a 2-year disease-free survival of 23%. Alvarnas et al. reported 15 patients with CNS disease (two primary CNS lymphoma and 13 secondary CNS lymphoma) treated with high-dose chemotherapy and hematopoietic transplantation [73], most of whom did not have active CNS disease at the time of transplantation. Five-year event-free and overall survival were 46% and 41% respectively [73]. Kasamon et al. reviewed 37 patients with DLBCL and T-cell lymphoblastic lymphoma with CNS involvement. CNS disease was treated into remission, and then the patients underwent autologous or allogeneic blood or bone marrow transplant. The 5-year actuarial event-free survival was 36% and overall survival was 39% [69].

Aggressive treatment to induce a CNS remission prior to transplantation is necessary to achieve optimal clinical outcomes [69]. A treatment strategy that may be beneficial in obtaining remission in the CNS is enhanced delivery of methotrexate-based chemotherapy in conjunction with osmotic opening of the blood-brain barrier. This technique of enhanced chemotherapy delivery to the CNS has been previously described [15, 74]. The goal of this treatment modality is to enhance delivery of therapeutic agents to the brain resulting in improved treatment outcome, while preserving neurocognitive function and quality of life [15].

Clinical results using osmotic blood-brain barrier disruption (BBBD) include a series of 74 patients with primary CNS lymphoma treated with methotrexate-based chemotherapy with BBBD [75, 76]. In this series the CR rate was 65% (48 patients), and 75% (36 patients) were in complete remission at one year. The estimated 5-year overall survival was 42%, with median survival of 40.7 months [75]. Kraemer et al. reported a statistically significant relationship between dose intensity and improved survival in this series of patients treated with BBBD [76]. This treatment modality offers an approach to achieving disease remission in the CNS, can be cycled with systemic treatment (intrathecal and intravenous chemotherapy), then consolidated with high-dose chemotherapy and hematopoietic stem call transplantation. This combined approach offers cycled dose intensive treatment to both CNS and systemic disease.

Multi-specialty collaboration is important in systematically studying and managing CNS relapse. At the time of this writing, analysis and reporting of a retrospective review of disease characteristics and clinical outcomes in patients with isolated brain parenchyma involvement of non-Hodgkin's lymphoma, is in progress [58]. The case series review was assembled by IPCG investigators. Just as international collaborative group retrospective series are important in compiling information on disease characteristics and treatment outcomes, multi-center prospective studies are needed to improve clinical outcomes in CNS relapse. Knowledge gained from systematic data collection and analysis, improved diagnostic strategies for early identification of CNS metastases, and aggressive intervention aimed at both CNS and systemic non-Hodgkin's lymphoma disease sites, will improve clinical outcomes.

The clinical impact of CNS metastases has become increasingly important as new treatment strategies better control systemic disease and improve survival of patients with non-Hodgkin's lymphoma. The occurrence of CNS relapse in patients with chronic myeloid leukemia treated on imatinib mesylate protocols has been reported by Leis at al [16]. With the addition of the monoclonal antibody rituximab to CHOP chemotherapy (R-CHOP) and improved survival rates in non-Hodgkin's lymphoma, CNS relapse may occur with increased frequency, perhaps because of poor penetration of rituximab across the blood-brain barrier [30].

References

1. van Besien K, Ha CS, Murphy S et al. Risk factors, treatment, and outcome of central nervous system recurrence in adults with intermediate-grade and immunoblastic lymphoma. Blood 1998; 91:1178–1184.
2. Bierman P, Giglio P. Diagnosis and treatment of central nervous system involvement in non-Hodgkin's lymphoma. Hematol Oncol Clin N Am 2005; 19:597–609.
3. Lister TA, Coiffier B, Armitage JO. Non-Hodgkin's lymphoma. In Abeloff MD, Armitage JO, Niederhuber JE, Kastan MB, McKenna WG, editors. Clinical oncology. Philadelphia: Elsevier, 2004:3015–3076.

4. Montoto S, Lister TA. Secondary central nervous system lymphoma: risk factors and prophylaxis. Hematol Oncol Clin N Am 2005; 19:751–763.
5. Grier J, Batchelor T. Metastatic neurologic complications of non-Hodgkin's lymphoma. Curr Oncol Rep 2005; 7:55–60.
6. Steinherz PG. CNS leukemia: problem of diagnosis, treatment, and outcome. J Clin Oncol 1995; 13:310–313.
7. Pinkel D, Woo S. Prevention and treatment of meningeal leukemia in children. Blood 1994; 84:355–366.
8. Bunn PA, Schein PS, Banks PM et al. Central nervous system complications in patients with diffuse histiocytic and undifferentiated lymphoma: leukemia revisited. Blood 1976; 47:3–10.
9. Kantarjian HM, Faderl S. Acute lymphoid leukemia in adults. In Abeloff MD, Armitage JO, Niederhuber JE, Kastan MB, McKenna WG, editors. Clinical oncology. Philadelphia:Elsevier, 2004:2793–2824.
10. Stewart DJ, Keating MJ, McCredie KB et al. Natural history of central nervous system acute leukemia in adults. Cancer 1981; 47:184–196.
11. Hegde U, Filie A, Little RF et al. High incidence of occult leptomeningeal disease detected by flow cytometry in newly diagnosed aggressive B-cell lymphomas at risk for central nervous system involvement: the role of flow cytometry versus cytology. Blood 2005; 105:496–502.
12. Kesari S, Batchelor TT. Leptomeningeal metastases. Neurol Clin N Am 2003; 21:25–66.
13. Sheehan T, Cuthbert RJG, Parker AC. Central nervous system involvement in haematological malignancies. Clin Lab Haemat 1989; 11:331–338.
14. Abbott NJ, Romero IA. Transporting therapeutics across the blood-brain barrier. Mol Med Today 1996; 2:106–113.
15. Kroll RA, Neuwelt EA. Outwitting the blood-brain barrier for therapeutic purposes: osmotic opening and other means. Neurosurgery 1998; 42:1083–1100.
16. Leis JF, Stepan DE, Curtin PT et al. Central nervous system failure in patients with chronic myelogenous leukemia lymphoid blast crisis and Philadelphia chromosome positive acute lymphoblastic leukemia treated with imatinib (STI-571). Leuk Lymphoma 2004; 45:695–698.
17. Petzer AL, Gunsilius E, Hayes M et al. Low concentrations of STI571 in the cerebrospinal fluid: a case report. Br J Haematol 2002; 117:623–625.
18. Takayama N, Sato N, O'Brien SG et al. Imatinib mesylate has limited activity against the central nervous system involvement of Philadelphia chromosome-positive acute lymphoblastic leukemia due to poor penetration into cerebrospinal fluid. Br J Hematol 2002; 119:106–108.
19. Traweek ST. Nervous system involvement by lymphoma, leukemia and other hematopoietic cell proliferations. In Bigner DD, McLendon RE, Bruner JM, editors. Russell and Rubinstein's pathology of tumors of the nervous system. London: Oxford University Press, 1998:195–237.

20. Ahn JY, Kwon SO, Shin MS et al. Meningeal chloroma (granulocytic sarcoma) in acute lymphoblastic leukemia mimicking a falx meningioma. J Neurooncol 2002; 60:31–35.

21. Lee S-H, Park J, Hwang S-K. Isolated recurrence of intracerebral granulocytic sarcoma in acute lymphoblastic leukemia: a case report. J Neurooncol 2006; 80:101–104.

22. Neiman RS, Barcos M, Berard C et al. Granulocytic sarcoma: a clinicopathologic study of 61 biopsied cases. Cancer 1981; 48:1426–1437.

23. Jaffe ES. The World Health Organization classification of hematologic malignancies. In: Abeloff MD, Armitage JO, Niederhuber JE, Kastan MB, McKenna WG, editors. Clinical oncology. Philadelphia: Elsevier, 2004: 2723–2730.

24. Harris NL, Jaffe ES, Stein H et al. A revised European-American classification of lymphoid neoplasms: a proposal from the International Lymphoma Study Group. Blood 1994; 84:1361–1392.

25. Jaffe ES, Harris NL, Stein H et al. Pathology and Genetics of Tumours of Hematopoietic and Lymphoid Tissues. Lyon, France: IARC Press, 2001.

26. Sehn LH, Berry B, Chhanabhai M et al. Revised international prognostic index (R-IPI) is a better predictor of outcome than the standard IPI for patients with diffuse large B-cell lymphoma treated with R-CHOP. Blood e-pub Nov. 14, 2006; doi 10.1182/blood-2006–08–038257.

27. Coiffier B, Lepage E, Briere J et al. CHOP chemotherapy plus rituximab compared with CHOP alone in elderly patients with diffuse large B-cell lymphoma. N Engl J Med 2002; 346:235–242.

28. Feugier P, Van Hoof A, Sebban C et al. Long-term results of the R-CHOP study in the treatment of elderly patients with diffuse large B-cell lymphoma: a study of the Group d'Etude des Lymphomes de l'Adulte. J Clin Oncol 2005; 23:4117–4126.

29. Sehn LH, Donaldson J, Chhanabhai M et al. Introduction of combined CHOP plus rituximab therapy dramatically improved outcome of diffuse large B-cell lymphoma in British Columbia. J Clin Oncol 2005; 23:5027–5033.

30. Harjunpaa A, Wiklund T, Collan et al. Complement activation in circulation and central nervous system after rituximab (anti-CD20) treatment of B-cell lymphoma. Leuk Lymphoma 2001; 42:731–738.

31. Feugier P, Virion JM, Tilly H et al. Incidence and risk factors for central nervous system occurrence in elderly patients with diffuse large-B-cell lymphoma: influence of rituximab. Ann Oncol 2004; 15:129–133.

32. Rubenstein JL, Combs D, Rosenberg J et al. Rituximab therapy for CNS lymphomas: targeting the leptomeningeal compartment. Blood 2003; 101: 466–468.

33. Bollen ELEM, Brouwer RE, Hamers S et al. Central nervous system relapse in non-Hodgkin lymphoma: a single-center study of 532 patients. Arch Neurol 1997; 54:854–859.

34. Ersboll J, Schultz HB, Thomsen BLR et al. Meningeal involvement in non-Hodgkin's lymphoma: symptoms, incidence, risk factors and treatment. Scand J Haematol 1985; 35:487–496.
35. Hollender A, Kvaloy S, Nome O et al. Central nervous system involvement following diagnosis of non-Hodgkin's lymphoma: a risk model. Ann Oncol 2002; 13:1099–1107.
36. Batchelor T, Leahy N, Kaufman D. High-dose methotrexate for isolated central nervous system relapse in patients with testicular non-Hodgkin's lymphoma. Clin Lymphoma 2001; 2:116–119.
37. Montserrat E, Bosch F, Lopez-Guillermo A et al. CNS involvement in mantle-cell lymphoma. J Clin Oncol 1996; 14:941–944.
38. Zucca E, Conconi A, Mughal TI et al. Patterns of outcome and prognostic factors in primary large-cell lymphoma of the testis in a survey by the international extranodal lymphoma study group. J Clin Oncol 2003; 21:20–27.
39. Spectre G, Gural A, Amir G et al. Central nervous system involvement in indolent lymphomas. Ann Oncol 2005; 16:450–454.
40. Zinzani PL, Magagnoli M, Frezza G et al. Isolated central nervous system relapse in aggressive non-Hodgkin's lymphoma: the Bologna experience. Leuk Lymphoma 1999; 32:571–576.
41. Bokstein F, Lossos A, Lossos IS et al. Central nervous system relapse of systemic non-Hodgkin's Lymphoma: results of treatment based on high-dose methotrexate combination chemotherapy. Leuk Lymphoma 2002; 43:587–593.
42. Haioun C, Besson C, Lepage E et al. Incidence and risk factors of central nervous system relapse in histologically aggressive non-Hodgkin's lymphoma uniformly treated and receiving intrathecal central nervous system prophylaxis: A GELA study on 974 patients. Ann Oncol 2000; 11:685–690.
43. Keldsen N, Michalski W, Bentzen SM et al. Risk factors for central nervous system involvement in non-Hodgkin's lymphoma. Acta Oncol 1996; 35: 703–708.
44. Bashir RM, Bierman PJ, Vose JM et al. Central nervous system involvement in patients with diffuse aggressive non-Hodgkin's lymphoma. Am J Clin Oncol 1991; 14:478–482.
45. Jahnke K, Thiel E, Martus P et al. Retrospective study of prognostic factors in non-Hodgkin lymphoma secondarily involving the central nervous system. Ann Hematol 2006; 85:45–50.
46. Boehme V, Zeynalova S, Kloess M et al. Incidence and risk factors of central nervous system recurrence in aggressive lymphoma: a survey of 1693 patients treated in protocols of the German high-grade non-Hodgkin's lymphoma study group (DSHNHL). Ann Oncol, e-pub October 3, 2006, doi:10.1093/annonc/mdl327.
47. Cairncross JG, Posner JB. Neurological complications of malignant lymphoma. In: Vinken PJ, Bruyn GW, editors. Handbook of clinical neurology. Amsterdam: Elsevier North-Holland Biomedical Press, 1980:27–61.

48. Hoster HA, Dratman MB, Craver LF et al. Hodgkin's disease, 1832–1947. Cancer Res 1948; 8:1–78.
49. Recht L, Mrugala M. Neurologic complications of hematologic neoplasms. Neurol Clin N Am 2003; 21:87–105.
50. Buckstein R, Lim W, Franssen E et al. CNS prophylaxis and treatment in non-Hodgkin's lymphoma: variation in practice and lessons from the literature. Leuk Lymphoma 2003; 44:955–962.
51. Tomita N, Kodama F, Kanamori H et al. Prophylactic intrathecal methotrexate and hydrocortisone reduces central nervous system recurrence and improves survival in aggressive non-Hodgkin's lymphoma. Cancer 2002; 95:576–580.
52. Levitt LJ, Dawson DM, Rosenthal DS et al. CNS involvement in the non-Hodgkin's lymphomas. Cancer 1980; 45:545–552.
53. Litam JP, Cabanillas F, Smith TL et al. Central nervous system relapse in malignant lymphomas: risk factors and implications for prophylaxis. Blood 1979; 54:1249–1257.
54. Chamberlain MC. Leptomeningeal metastases: a review of evaluation and treatment. J Neurooncol 1998; 37:271–284.
55. Siegal T. Leptomeningeal metastases: rationale for systemic chemotherapy or what is the role of intra-CSF chemotherapy? J Neurooncol 1998; 38: 151–157.
56. Recht L, Straus DJ, Cirrincione C et al. Central nervous system metastases from Non-Hodgkin's lymphoma: treatment and prophylaxis. Am J Med 1988; 84:425–435.
57. Mackintosh FR, Colby TV, Podolsky WJ et al. Central nervous system involvement in non-Hodgkin's Lymphoma: an analysis of 105 cases. Cancer 1982; 49:586–595.
58. Doolittle ND, Abrey L, Shenkier T et al. Isolated brain parenchyma relapse of non-Hodgkin's Lymphoma: a descriptive analysis from the International Primary CNS Lymphoma Collaborative Group (IPCG). Blood 2006; 108:574a (abstract #2026).
59. Wong ET, Portlock CS, O'Brien JP et al. Chemosensitive epidural spinal cord disease in non-Hodgkin's lymphoma. Neurology 1996; 46:1543–1547.
60. van Oostenbrugge RJ, Twijnstra A. Presenting features and value of diagnostic procedures in leptomeningeal metastases. Neurology 1999; 53:382–385.
61. DeAngelis LM, Cairncross JG. A better way to find tumor in the CSF? Neurology 2002; 58:339–340.
62. Ferreri AJM, Abrey LE, Blay J-V et al. Summary statement on primary central nervous system lymphomas from the eighth international conference on malignant lymphoma, Lugano, Switzerland, June 12 to 15, 2002. J Clin Oncol 2003; 21:2407–2414.
63. Tomita N, Kodama F, Kanamori H et al. Secondary central nervous system lymphoma. Int J Hematol 2006; 84:128–135.

64. Colocci N, Glantz M, Recht L. Prevention and treatment of central nervous system involvement by non-Hodgkin's lymphoma: a review of the literature. Semin Neurol 2004; 24:395–404.
65. Gavrilovic IT, Hormigo A, Yahalom J et al. Long-term follow-up of high-dose methotrexate-based therapy with and without whole brain irradiation for newly diagnosed primary CNS lymphoma. J Clin Oncol 2006; 24: 4570–4574.
66. Glantz MJ, Cole BF, Recht L et al. High-dose intravenous methotrexate for patients with nonleukemic leptomeningeal cancer: Is intrathecal chemotherapy necessary? J Clin Oncol 1998; 16:1561–1567.
67. Bleyer WA. Neurologic sequelae of methotrexate and ionizing radiation: a new classification. Cancer Treatment Reports 1981; 65(Suppl 1):89–98.
68. Young RC, Howser DM, Anderson T et al. Central nervous system complications of non-Hodgkin's Lymphoma. Am J Med 1979; 66:435–443.
69. Kasaman YL, Jones RJ, Piantadosi S et al. High-dose chemotherapy and blood or marrow transplantation for non-Hodgkin lymphoma with central nervous system involvement. Biol Blood Marrow Transplant 2005; 11:93–100.
70. van Besien K, Forman A, Champlin R. Central nervous system relapse of lymphoid malignancies in adults: the role of high-dose chemotherapy. Ann Oncol 1997; 8:515–524.
71. Williams CD, Pearce R, Taghipour G et al. Autologous bone marrow transplantation for patients with non-Hodgkin's lymphoma and CNS involvement: those transplanted with active CNS disease have a poor outcome: a report by the European Bone Marrow Transplant Lymphoma Registry. J Clin Oncol 1994; 12: 2415–2422.
72. van Besien K, Przepiorka D, Mehra R et al. Impact of preexisiting CNS involvement on the outcome of bone marrow transplantation in adult hematologic malignancies. J Clin Oncol 1996; 14:3036–3042.
73. Alvarnas JC, Negrin RS, Horning SJ et al. High-dose therapy with hematopoietic cell transplantation for patients with central nervous system involvement by non-Hodgkin's lymphoma. Biol Blood Marrow Transplant 2000; 6:352–358.
74. Neuwelt EA, Goldman DL, Dahlborg SA et al. Primary CNS lymphoma treated with osmotic blood-brain barrier disruption: prolonged survival and preservation of cognitive function. J Clin Oncol 1991; 9:1580–1590.
75. McAllister LD, Doolittle ND, Guastadisegni PE et al. Cognitive outcomes and long-term follow-up results after enhanced chemotherapy delivery for primary central nervous system lymphoma. Neurosurgery 2000; 46: 51–61.
76. Kraemer DF, Fortin D, Doolittle ND et al. Association of total dose intensity of chemotherapy in primary central nervous system lymphoma (human non-acquired immunodeficiency syndrome) and survival. Neurosurgery 2001; 48:1033–1041.

10. Chemotherapy for Brain Metastases: Breast, Gynecologic and Non-Melanoma Skin Malignancies

Gaurav D. Shah, MD and Lauren E. Abrey, MD

Introduction

Greater than one-half of all intracranial tumors in adults represent metastases from disseminated systemic malignancies. Abundant class I evidence has been accumulated for the past two decades that demonstrates improved survival and quality of life with surgical resection or SRS for appropriate patients. In some tumor types, WBRT can effectively treat, prevent and/or delay recurrences and improve survival as well. However, several factors may preclude either surgery or radiation therapy (e.g., number of metastases, co-existing medical or neurological conditions) and in such patients the mainstay of treatment is chemotherapy or other biologic targeted therapy.

Solid tumor malignancies that commonly metastasize to the brain include lung cancer (30 to 60% of all brain metastases), breast cancer, melanoma, renal cell cancer, colorectal cancer, germ cell tumors, and systemic Non-Hodgkin's lymphoma (NHL). However, this list is by no means exhaustive, and access to the lymphovascular space substantially increases this risk for virtually any solid tumor type.

In this chapter, we review chemotherapy options for brain metastases from breast, gynecologic and skin cancers. It should be noted that in most cases, brain metastases have been evaluated only in the broader context of treatment for systemically disseminated disease; however, we review brain-targeted treatment where available.

Our review of gynecologic malignancies includes ovarian and fallopian tube cancer, endometrial cancer, cervical cancer, germ cell tumors and gestational trophoblastic disease (GTD). Our review of skin cancers will address non-melanomatous malignancies.

Responsiveness to Chemotherapy

The responsiveness of brain metastases to chemotherapy depends largely on two factors; limitations imposed by the blood-brain barrier, and tumor chemosensitivity.

A common misconception is that the blood-brain barrier remains intact in brain malignancies (primary or secondary) and, therefore, acts as a significant obstacle to chemotherapy efficacy. Although some hydrophilic drugs and large molecules are prevented from entering normal brain tissue, contrast enhancement on MRI in high-grade primary gliomas, lymphomas, and metastases point to a clearly, if partially disrupted blood-brain barrier. Furthermore, systemic chemotherapy has been demonstrated to lead to objective responses in brain metastases (see below), thus further supporting evidence for a disrupted barrier. It should be noted that the use of corticosteroids may restore an otherwise disrupted blood-brain barrier and should, therefore, be used sparingly during chemotherapeutic treatment.

There is no *a priori* reason to believe that brain metastases differ in chemosensitivity from other systemic metastases, and in fact response rates tend to be comparable. However, published phase II and III studies of chemotherapy in brain metastases have been less than illuminating for several reasons. First, brain metastases often occur late in the disease course, at a time when previously sensitive tumor cells have already become resistant and/or more aggressive. Second, systemic disease progression is often debilitating and specific treatment of brain metastases is limited by the patient's poor medical and/or performance status. Finally, many well-designed studies fail to stratify by disease type; the literature is therefore ripe with discussions of terms such as "poor prognosis brain metastases" and "favorable prognosis brain metastases."

Breast Cancer

An estimated 170,000 new cases of breast cancer are diagnosed yearly in the United States. Although this incidence has been rising over several years largely due to early detection, the mortality rate has been decreasing slightly, pointing to progress in effective therapy.

Brain metastases from breast cancer have been associated with several negative prognostic factors including younger age, premenopausal status, infiltrating ductal carcinoma histology (IDC), estrogen receptor (ER) and progesterone receptor (PR) negativity, low Bcl-2 expression, high proportion of S-phase, aneuploidy, and altered p53. HER2/neu status has not been shown to be a prognostic factor [1].

Brain metastases from breast cancer are being reported with increasing frequency. This apparent increase in prevalence at least partly stems from effective systemic therapy with trastuzumab in HER2/neu positive patients, and concomitant lack of central nervous system (CNS) penetration of this large molecule. Furthermore, improved visceral disease control with trastuzumab as well as other chemotherapy agents is associated with improved survival and eventual onset of CNS disease [2, 3].

Metastatic breast cancer is relatively responsive to chemotherapy with reported response rates to combination doxorubicin/cyclophosphamide/taxane therapy upwards of 58% [4–6]. Trastuzumab alone is known to have a response rate of 19–26% in patients with over-expression of HER2/neu [7, 8], and hormonal therapy alone is also associated with a 33% response rate [9].

These same agents generally have poor CNS penetration across an intact blood-brain barrier, but objective responses have been seen in brain metastases, again supporting at least partial barrier disruption in brain metastases. Table 1 summarizes the literature on breast cancer chemotherapy in brain metastases.

Rosner et al.'s study is the most comprehensive prospective assessment of brain metastasis response to various standard regimens approved in metastatic breast cancer. Of the 100 patients evaluated, 63 had received prior adjuvant chemotherapy.

Table 1. Chemotherapy for breast cancer metastasizing to the brain

Study	Agent(s)	N	Objective Response (CR+PR)	Other data
Rosner et al. [10]	CFP	52	52%	Medial overall survival (OS)
	CFP-MV	35	54%	for CR=39.5m; PR=10.5m;
	MVP	7	43%	non-resp = 1.5m. 37%
	AC	6	17%	response rate to different rx upon relapse
Boogerd et al. [11]	CMF or CAF	20 2	59%	Median OS = 6 months
Cocconi et al. [12]	platinum + etoposide	22	55% (23% CR, 32% PR)	OS = 14m
Zulkowski et al. [13]	bendamustine	1	PR	Case report
Wang et al. [14]	Capecitabine	1	PR	Case report
Siegelmann-Danieli et al. [15]	Capecitabine	1	CR	Case report
Abrey et al. [16]	Temozolomide	10	0	TTP = 2.7 months
Christodoulou et al. [17]	Temozolomide	4	0	Heavily pre-treated patients
Lassman et al. [18]	High-dose M	29	28%	OS = 20 weeks
Lin et al. [19]	Lapatinib	39	5%	Trastuzumab-refractory Her-2/Neu + patients. additional minor response in 3%, and SD in 13%

*C = cyclophosphamide; F = 5-fluorouracil; P = prednisone; M = methotrexate; V = vincristine; A = doxorubicin (Adriamycin); TTP = time to tumor progression; CR = complete response; PR = partial response

Ten achieved a CR, 40 a PR, and another nine had stable disease (SD). It is interesting to note that the best responses (upwards of 50%) were achieved using regimens that are not routinely used in oncological care in the United States though often employed in Canada and Europe. Survival was significantly improved with the use of chemotherapy [10].

Boogerd et al., prospectively evaluated a total of 22 patients with brain metastases from breast cancer treated with either CMF or CAF. Seven had already received prior chemotherapy. The objective response rate was 59%, including in four of seven patients who had previously been treated with surgery or radiation for brain metastases [11].

Cisplatin and etoposide have also been evaluated in this setting with relatively promising results. Of 22 patients, five (23%) achieved a CR and seven (32%) a PR, for a total response rate of 55%. Furthermore, median duration of sustained response was approximately nine months, with a median survival of almost 14 months [12].

In a study designed to evaluate brain metastases from several malignancies, Abrey et al. evaluated 10 patients with breast cancer. Although there were no objective responses, four (40%) had SD; median time to tumor progression was 2.7 months [16].

Smaller studies and case reports have given further support to the use of chemotherapy in brain metastases using bendamustine and capecitabine. Recently, Lassman et al. demonstrated a 28% response rate to high-dose (3.5 g/m^2) methotrexate [18].

HER2/neu over-expressing patients historically have had an inferior overall prognosis before the advent of the targeted antibody trastuzumab. However, even with single agent trastuzumab, once the breast cancer has progressed to stage IV, response rates are lower than those achieved with chemotherapy. Furthermore, trastuzumab is a large molecule with little if any CNS penetration; thus even the 19–26% response rate noted above is not likely reproducible in brain metastases.

Improved results have been reported with lapatinib, an oral, smaller multi-targeted antibody that works against the HER2/neu surface protein as well as against epidermal growth factor receptor (EGFR). In a preliminary report of 39 women who developed brain metastases while receiving trastuzumab, there were two partial and one minor response; in addition, five patients had stable disease for four months or longer.

A phase I study of lapatinib dosed from 500 to 1,600 mg demonstrated four PRs out of 30 breast cancer patients who overexpressed HER2/neu. These patients were heavily pre-treated and deemed refractory to trastuzumab [20]. Preliminary data from a phase II trial of 39 patients who had developed brain metastases while on trastuzumab revealed two PRs with lapatinib 1500 mg daily, and one minor response by RECIST criteria, while an additional five maintained SD for at least 16 weeks [21].

Lapatinib has also been combined with capecitabine in a phase III trial recently presented at ASCO [22]. The study was terminated early after enrollment of 392 patients when time to tumor progression (TTP) supported combination lapatinib + capecitabine over capecitabine alone. Lapatinib was associated with fewer brain metastases as the initial site of disease progression further demonstrating its relative efficacy in CNS. However, at the most recent follow-up, no improvement in survival was detected.

To summarize, there are no clear-cut recommendations for the chemotherapeutic management of brain metastases from breast cancer, and the choice of drug needs to take into consideration prior treatment regimens as well as toxicity profiles. Combination therapy with cyclophosphamide, 5-FU, methotrexate and cisplatin-based regimens seems appropriate as first-line management, with consideration of lapatinib in combination with capecitabine for HER2/neu over-expressing patients. Ongoing trials with novel agents, such as the non-taxane microtubule inhibitor patupilone, are underway.

Gynecologic Malignancies

Approximately 13% of the 650,000 yearly cases of malignancies diagnosed in women are gynecologic in origin. However, the incidence of brain metastases from gynecologic cancers is closer to 1% or less, with only 2% of all brain metastases arising from gynecologic malignancies. This number may be increasing due to increase survival and late development of CNS disease.

Ovarian Cancer (Epithelial)

Brain metastases from epithelial ovarian cancer are rare and represent a late stage of disease. Optimally, debulked ovarian cancer is routinely treated with adjuvant chemotherapy. The most common regimen used in clinical practice is carboplatin plus paclitaxel.

The importance of chemotherapy in the management of brain metastases from ovarian cancer is controversial since concomitant disease is usually present at other non-CNS sites as well. The standard of care for brain metastases is surgery and/or SRS (if possible) followed by WBRT with chemotherapy for any remaining systemic disease. The choice of chemotherapy often depends on prior regimens as well as elapsed time since last chemotherapy administration [23].

Chemotherapy has been evaluated in the context of surgical management for brain metastases from ovarian cancer. A retrospective review of 104 such patients revealed a median time to development of brain metastases from ovarian cancer diagnosis of 19.5 months. The majority of patients had radiation therapy and/or surgery incorporated into their management. In addition to surgery, chemotherapy was found to be a strong independent predictor of survival with cisplatin-based therapy associated with markedly improved survival (13 months versus five months, P=0.002) [24].

Carboplatin-based therapy has been evaluated independent of surgery or radiation and was found to be associated with objective responses of brain metastases from epithelial ovarian cancer. Vlasveld et al. have described a CR [25], while Cooper et al. described one CR and two PRs with survival ranging from 11 to 25 months in three women treated with carboplatin [26]. A combination of carboplatin and paclitaxel induced a sustained CR in a patient with multiple brain metastases who had been previously treated with the same regimen in an adjuvant setting; her eventual demise was, however, due to leptomeningeal progression [27].

Cisplatin has never been tested alone, but in one case report a combination of gemcitabine with cisplatin was found to help induce a CR when used in conjunction with WBRT as well as with 5-FU for three subsequent recurrences [28].

Fallopian Tube Cancer

Malignancies of the fallopian tube are rare, accounting for less than 1% of gyneco-logic malignancies. They are managed in a method similar to epithelial ovarian cancer. Brain metastases have been described only in case reports, but the only report of chemotherapeutic management described a complete remission maintained for 36 months after surgical resection and combination cisplatin with cyclophos-phamide [29].

Germ Cell Tumors of the Ovary

Malignant ovarian germ cell tumors include dysgerminomas, endodermal sinus carcinomas, immature teratomas, ovarian choriocarcinomas, and mixed histologies. The general guidelines for treatment of these tumors are identical to those for epithelial ovarian cancer. However, germ cell tumors are extremely chemosensitive to platinum-based therapy, and unlike other solid tumors, brain metastases from ovarian germ cell tumors can be eradicated with chemotherapy [30].

The standard chemotherapy regimen for both dysgerminomas and non-dysgerminomas is BEP (bleomycin, etoposide, cisplatin). For advanced disease involving the brain, four cycles are recommended for dysgerminomas and six for non-dysgerminomas. In one study of 26 advanced dysgerminoma patients treated with BEP for three to six cycles, a remarkable 25 (96%) remained disease-free at a follow up time of 89 months, while the remaining patient had a second primary in the other ovary and was cured completely after surgical resection [31]. This high response rate is not limited to dysgerminomas. A case report of a young woman with ovarian mixed germ cell tumor with pulmonary metastases, and an occipital brain metastasis, describes CRs in both sites after surgical resection and several cycles of chemotherapy including combination etoposide, methotrexate, actinomycin-D, cyclophosphamide and vincristine (EMA/CO), with no evidence of disease recurrence at 98 months [32].

Gestational Trophoblastic Disease

Gestational trophoblastic disease (GTD), also known as choriocarcinoma, has become one of the most eradicable oncologic diseases since the incorporation of methotrexate into standard chemotherapy regimens. The development of brain metastases is considered a poor prognostic indicator for GTD, although complete responses are not uncommon.

There are two standard approaches to the management of CNS metastases from GTD. One approach incorporates intrathecal methotrexate into standard EMA/CO therapy, and the other calls for cranial irradiation. Both approaches are associated with promising results for long-term survival of patients who had CNS metastases at diagnosis, but not for those with recurrent brain metastases despite prior therapy.

Rustin et al. [33] evaluated 25 patients with brain metastases from GTD treated with EMA/CO, with an intravenous methotrexate dose of 1 g/m^2 and 12.5 mg intrathecal methotrexate instituted into the regimen. Thirteen of 18 (72%) patients who had CNS metastases at presentation and were treated with EMA/CO remained disease-free at a median follow-up of 33 months. An additional two of seven patients who had developed CNS metastases despite prior EMA/CO responded to surgery and further chemotherapy (methotrexate and actinomycin in one case; mercaptopurine in the other).

A United Kingdom-based retrospective life-table analysis of 69 patients with brain metastases from GTD, treated with an EMA/CO regimen that also incorporated intrathecal methotrexate, projected a vastly improved long-term survival (49%) for patients who had presented with brain metastases over those who developed them despite prior therapy (6% survival) [34]. Cranial irradiation was used selectively in these patients.

Similar results are seen when cranial irradiation is instituted into treatment planning for all patients without concomitant intrathecal methotrexate. Evans et al. [35] evaluated 42 patients with GTD metastatic to the CNS treated with 3000 cGY WBRT in addition to methotrexate, actinomycin-D and chlorambucil or an alternate etoposide-based regimen. Seventy-five percent of patients with brain metastases at diagnosis, 38% with brain metastases despite prior therapy, and 0% who developed brain metastases during therapy were alive at one year.

Either treatment approach may be employed (EMA/CO plus either intrathecal methotrexate or WBRT), and the choice of approach should depend on long-term toxicity.

Endometrial Cancer

Brain metastases from endometrial cancer are exceedingly rare and have been evaluated less than in ovarian cancer. When present, a multimodal treatment approach is usually indicated including adjuvant chemotherapy with single or combination agents often including doxorubicin and/or cisplatin/carboplatin. Survival of greater than 30 months has been reported [36].

Although no studies have specifically examined chemotherapy targeted against brain metastases from endometrial cancer, short-duration systemic disease response rates of 36 to 67% have been reported with various combinations of cisplatin/doxorubicin/cyclophosphamide, and responses of 20 to 37% have been reported with single-agent doxorubicin, cisplatin, carboplatin, topotecan, and paclitaxel. The specific addition of paclitaxel to combination therapy has been associated with a tangible survival benefit [37]. No trial has specifically addressed clinical or radiographic changes in brain metastases during therapy. It should be noted that patients with recurrent serous papillary or clear cell endometrial histologies can rarely be cured, and the approach in such a setting is more similar to epithelial ovarian cancer, with combination paclitaxel and carboplatin being commonly employed. Finally, the additional of megestrol acetate (Megace) as hormonal therapy may be of benefit as well.

Cervical Cancer

Like endometrial cancer, cervical cancer metastasis to the brain is rare. The incidence of squamous cell carcinoma and adenocarcinoma histologies is similar. In one retrospective study of primary irradiated cervical cancer patients, only 18 of 322 patients with metastatic disease had brain involvement, and a few reported cases have been treated successfully with surgery and/or radiation therapy [38–40]. However, the lack of data renders it difficult to specifically address chemotherapy for brain metastases from cervical cancer, and the standard of care involves a combination of systemic chemotherapy (single agent platinum or a platinum-based doublet combination regimen, e.g., cisplatin + ifosfamide or carboplatin + paclitaxel), surgery and radiation therapy.

Cutaneous Malignancies (Excluding Melanoma)

Cutaneous Squamous Cell and Basal Cell Carcinoma

To our knowledge, only one case of hematogenous spread of cutaneous squamous cell carcinoma to the brain has been reported to be successfully treated with resection and WBRT with no additional chemotherapy [41]. A fatal direct spread to the brain has also been described [42].

To our knowledge, no cases of basal cell carcinoma metastatic to the brain have ever been reported.

Merkel Cell Carcinoma

Merkel cell carcinoma (MCC) is an uncommon but aggressive cutaneous cancer arising from a neuroendocrine cell lineage and is associated with a higher risk of distant spread. Incorporating their own results into an extensive review of the literature, Tai et al. found a 75% response rate (35% CR) to a combination regimen of cisplatin + doxorubicin or epirubicin + vincristine (CAV) with or without prednisone, and a 60% response rate (36% CR) to etoposide + cisplatin or carboplatin (considered the standard regimen for other neuroendocrine tumors such as small-cell lung cancer) [43]. Median survival, however, was limited to 22 months.

Development of brain metastasis significantly decreases survival in patients with MCC. The literature is limited to case reports of a total of 13 patients including those with hematogenous and direct spread (from scalp-based primaries) [44–47]. All patients were treated with surgical resection, cranial irradiation, and chemotherapy using one of the standard regimens. Most patients died within nine months of diagnosis of brain metastases.

Concluding Remarks

In this chapter we have summarized current chemotherapeutic options for patients with brain metastases from breast cancer, gynecologic cancers and non-melanomatous skin cancers. Most existing knowledge about brain metastases from these and other solid tumors (see Chapter 11) comes from studies of patients with widespread systemic metastases, since the CNS is rarely the sole site of metastases and is often a marker of late- or end-stage disease. In some cases such as breast cancer, modestly effective brain-targeted therapy has been developed (e.g., lapatinib). In most cases (with the exceptions of GTD and germ cell tumors), resorting to chemotherapy implies a lack of surgical options, thus precluding attempts at brain tissue analysis and other strategies that may eventually help identify effective therapy targeted against brain metastases. However, with clinical advances and growing availability of tumor analysis technologies such as comparative genomic hybridization (cGH), obtaining brain tissue as part of experimental protocols may become increasingly relevant. Until then, chemotherapeutic options derived from experience in systemic metastases will continue to be an important part of care for patients with brain metastases as well.

References

1. Tham YL, Sexton K, Kramer R, Hilsenbeck S, Elledge R. Primary breast cancer phenotypes associated with propensity for central nervous system metastases. Cancer 2006;107(4):696–704.
2. Bendell JC, Domchek SM, Burstein HJ, et al. Central nervous system metastases in women who receive trastuzumab-based therapy for metastatic breast carcinoma. Cancer 2003;97(12):2972–7.
3. van den Bent MJ. The role of chemotherapy in brain metastases. Eur J Cancer 2003;39(15):2114–20.

4. Gianni L, Munzone E, Capri G, et al. Paclitaxel by 3-hour infusion in combination with bolus doxorubicin in women with untreated metastatic breast cancer: high antitumor efficacy and cardiac effects in a dose-finding and sequence-finding study. J Clin Oncol 1995;13(11):2688–99.

5. Lluch A, Ojeda B, Colomer R, et al. Doxorubicin and paclitaxel in advanced breast carcinoma: importance of prior adjuvant anthracycline therapy. Cancer 2000;89(11):2169–75.

6. Bria E, Giannarelli D, Felici A, et al. Taxanes with anthracyclines as first-line chemotherapy for metastatic breast carcinoma. Cancer 2005;103(4):672–9.

7. Vogel CL, Cobleigh MA, Tripathy D, et al. Efficacy and safety of trastuzumab as a single agent in first-line treatment of HER2-overexpressing metastatic breast cancer. J Clin Oncol 2002;20(3):719–26.

8. Baselga J, Carbonell X, Castaneda-Soto NJ, et al. Phase II study of efficacy, safety, and pharmacokinetics of trastuzumab monotherapy administered on a 3-weekly schedule. J Clin Oncol 2005;23(10):2162–71.

9. Howell A, Robertson JF, Abram P, et al. Comparison of fulvestrant versus tamoxifen for the treatment of advanced breast cancer in postmenopausal women previously untreated with endocrine therapy: a multinational, double-blind, randomized trial. J Clin Oncol 2004;22(9):1605–13.

10. Rosner D, Nemoto T, Lane WW. Chemotherapy induces regression of brain metastases in breast carcinoma. Cancer 1986;58(4):832–9.

11. Boogerd W, Dalesio O, Bais EM, van der Sande JJ. Response of brain metastases from breast cancer to systemic chemotherapy. Cancer 1992;69(4): 972–80.

12. Cocconi G, Lottici R, Bisagni G, et al. Combination therapy with platinum and etoposide of brain metastases from breast carcinoma. Cancer investigation 1990;8(3–4):327–34.

13. Zulkowski K, Kath R, Semrau R, Merkle K, Hoffken K. Regression of brain metastases from breast carcinoma after chemotherapy with bendamustine. Journal of cancer research and clinical oncology 2002;128(2):111–3.

14. Wang ML, Yung WK, Royce ME, Schomer DF, Theriault RL. Capecitabine for 5-fluorouracil-resistant brain metastases from breast cancer. Am J Clin Oncol 2001;24(4):421–4.

15. Siegelmann-Danieli N, Stein M, Bar-Ziv J. Complete response of brain metastases originating in breast cancer to capecitabine therapy. Isr Med Assoc J 2003;5(11):833–4.

16. Abrey LE, Olson JD, Raizer JJ, et al. A phase II trial of temozolomide for patients with recurrent or progressive brain metastases. Journal of neurooncology 2001;53(3):259–65.

17. Christodoulou C, Bafaloukos D, Kosmidis P, et al. Phase II study of temozolomide in heavily pretreated cancer patients with brain metastases. Ann Oncol 2001;12(2):249–54.

18. Lassman AB, Abrey LE, Shah GD, et al. Systemic high-dose intravenous methotrexate for central nervous system metastases. Journal of neuro-oncology 2006;78(3):255–60.

19. Lin YC, Liu HE, Wang CH, et al. Clinical benefit and response in patients with gastric cancer to weekly 24-hour infusion of high-dose 5-fluorouracil (5-FU) and leucovorin (LV). Anticancer research 1999;19(6C):5615–20.

20. Burris HA, 3rd, Hurwitz HI, Dees EC, et al. Phase I safety, pharmacokinetics, and clinical activity study of lapatinib (GW572016), a reversible dual inhibitor of epidermal growth factor receptor tyrosine kinases, in heavily pretreated patients with metastatic carcinomas. J Clin Oncol 2005;23(23):5305–13.

21. Lin N, Carey L, Liu M, et al. Phase II trial of lapatinib for brain metastases in patients with HER2+ breast cancer. Presented at the American Society of Clinical Oncology meeting (abstract #503). Journal of Clinical Oncology 2006;24(18S).

22. Geyer C, Cameron D, Lindquist D, et al. A phase III, randomized open-label, Internationsl study comparing lapatinib and capecitabine versus capecitabine in women with refractory advanced or metastatic breast cancer (abstract). Data presented at the annual meeting of the American Society of Clinical Oncology, 2006. 2006.

23. Pectasides D, Pectasides M, Economopoulos T. Brain metastases from epithelial ovarian cancer: a review of the literature. The oncologist 2006;11(3):252–60.

24. McMeekin DS, Kamelle SA, Vasilev SA, et al. Ovarian cancer metastatic to the brain: what is the optimal management? Journal of surgical oncology 2001;78(3):194–200; discussion -1.

25. Vlasveld LT, Beynen JH, Boogerd W, Ten Bokkel Huinink WW, Rodenhuis S. Complete remission of brain metastases of ovarian cancer following high-dose carboplatin: a case report and pharmacokinetic study. Cancer chemotherapy and pharmacology 1990;25(5):382–3.

26. Cooper KG, Kitchener HC, Parkin DE. Cerebral metastases from epithelial ovarian carcinoma treated with carboplatin. Gynecologic oncology 1994;55(2):318–23.

27. Watanabe A, Shimada M, Kigawa J, et al. The benefit of chemotherapy in a patient with multiple brain metastases and meningitis carcinomatosa from ovarian cancer. International journal of clinical oncology/Japan Society of Clinical Oncology 2005;10(1):69–71.

28. Melichar B, Urminska H, Kohlova T, Nova M, Cesak T. Brain metastases of epithelial ovarian carcinoma responding to cisplatin and gemcitabine combination chemotherapy: a case report and review of the literature. Gynecologic oncology 2004;94(2):267–76.

29. Hidaka T, Nakamura T, Shima T, Sumiya S, Saito S. Cerebral metastasis from a primary adenocarcinoma of the fallopian tube. Gynecologic oncology 2004;95(1):260–3.

30. Lu KH, Gershenson DM. Update on the management of ovarian germ cell tumors. The Journal of reproductive medicine 2005;50(6):417–25.
31. Brewer M, Gershenson DM, Herzog CE, Mitchell MF, Silva EG, Wharton JT. Outcome and reproductive function after chemotherapy for ovarian dysgerminoma. J Clin Oncol 1999;17(9):2670–75.
32. Adcock LL, Oakley GJ. A pure brain metastasis of choriocarcinoma from a mixed germ cell tumor of the ovary. Gynecologic oncology 1997;64(2):252–5.
33. Rustin GJ, Newlands ES, Begent RH, Dent J, Bagshawe KD. Weekly alternating etoposide, methotrexate, and actinomycin/vincristine and cyclophosphamide chemotherapy for the treatment of CNS metastases of choriocarcinoma. J Clin Oncol 1989;7(7):900–3.
34. Athanassiou A, Begent RH, Newlands ES, Parker D, Rustin GJ, Bagshawe KD. Central nervous system metastases of choriocarcinoma. 23 years' experience at Charing Cross Hospital. Cancer 1983;52(9):1728–35.
35. Evans AC, Jr., Soper JT, Clarke-Pearson DL, Berchuck A, Rodriguez GC, Hammond CB. Gestational trophoblastic disease metastatic to the central nervous system. Gynecologic oncology 1995;59(2):226–30.
36. Lee WJ, Chen CH, Chow SN. Brain metastases from early stage endometrial carcinoma 8 years after primary treatment. Case report and review of the literature. Acta obstetricia et gynecologica Scandinavica 2006;85(7):890–1.
37. Fleming GF, Brunetto VL, Cella D, et al. Phase III trial of doxorubicin plus cisplatin with or without paclitaxel plus filgrastim in advanced endometrial carcinoma: a Gynecologic Oncology Group Study. J Clin Oncol 2004;22(11):2159–66.
38. Amita M, Sudeep G, Rekha W, Yogesh K, Hemant T. Brain metastasis from cervical carcinoma–a case report. MedGenMed 2005;7(1):26.
39. Gaussmann AB, Imhoff D, Lambrecht E, Menzel C, Mose S. Spontaneous remission of metastases of cancer of the uterine cervix. Onkologie 2006;29(4):159–61.
40. Nagar YS, Shah N, Rawat S, Kataria T. Intracranial metastases from adenocarcinoma of cervix: a case report. Int J Gynecol Cancer 2005;15(3):561–3.
41. Salvati M, Caroli E, Paone C, et al. Brain metastasis from cutaneous squamous cell carcinoma of the dorsum. Case report. Journal of neurosurgery 2005;102(6):1155–8.
42. Simon CD, Sims PJ, Elston DM. Fatal cutaneous squamous cell carcinoma with extension through the maxillary sinus and orbit into the brain. Cutis; cutaneous medicine for the practitioner 1999;63(6):341–3.
43. Tai PT, Yu E, Winquist E, et al. Chemotherapy in neuroendocrine/Merkel cell carcinoma of the skin: case series and review of 204 cases. J Clin Oncol 2000;18(12):2493–9.
44. Faye N, Lafitte F, Martin Duverneuil N, et al. Merkel cell tumor: report of two cases and review of the literature. Journal of neuroradiology 2005;32(2):138–41.

45. Barkdull GC, Healy JF, Weisman RA. Intracranial spread of Merkel cell carcinoma through intact skull. The Annals of otology, rhinology, and laryngology 2004;113(9):683–7.
46. Turgut M. Brain metastasis of Merkel cell carcinoma. Neurosurgical review 2002;25(1–2):113–4.
47. Ikawa F, Kiya K, Uozumi T, et al. Brain metastasis of Merkel cell carcinoma. Case report and review of the literature. Neurosurgical review 1999;22(1):54–7.

11. Chemotherapy for Brain Metastases due to Lung Cancer and Melanoma

Marc C Chamberlain, M.D.

Introduction

Several issues are pertinent to a discussion of chemotherapy for brain metastases (BM) [Table 1]. First and most important, there is a paucity of clinical trials with very few randomized trials [1–6]. The limited evidence supporting the use of chemotherapy for BM comes from nonrandomized, retrospective studies and case reports. Second, survival is often limited by death from systemic disease (approximately 30% of patients with BM die as a direct result of central nervous system disease). Patients with BM are heterogeneous and the importance of stratification for prognostic factors for example by way of the Radiation Treatment Oncology Group recursive portioning analysis (RTOG RPA) is often overlooked [7]. Third, how to measure efficacy has proven challenging as many studies report overall survival as a primary outcome [Table 2]. Survival is most often used as an outcome measure of chemotherapeutic response however in patients with BM this is unlikely to reflect chemotherapy efficacy. As mentioned above, the majority of patients with BM die of systemic disease progression. More relevant is radiographic response, duration of response, maintenance or improvement in neurologic function and quality of life. Fourth, the majority of patients with BM have in general been treated with at least one and often two or more prior chemotherapy regimens. Consequently, the systemic cancer has developed acquired chemotherapy resistance such that few active chemotherapy agents remain available for treatment. Lastly, the majority of BM-chemotherapy trials have evaluated a single chemotherapy regimen directed at multiple tumor histologies making determinations of responsiveness against specific tumor histology problematic.

Two factors influence the efficacy of chemotherapy in BM; the intrinsic chemosensitivity of the tumor and chemotherapy drug delivery. Parenchymal brain drug delivery is determined by drug properties such as lipophilicity, ionization state and molecular weight and by the blood brain barrier (BBB). Because the majority of chemotherapy agents with activity against systemic cancer are non-lipophilic

Table 1. Issues regarding the treatment of brain metastases with chemotherapy

- Blood-brain-barrier
- Prior treatment with acquisition of acquired drug resistance
- Few effective chemotherapy agents
- Concurrent systemic disease
- Heterogeneity of patient population
- Heterogeneity of tumor types enrolled
- Measurement of efficacy
- Interpretation of the litrature

i.e. water soluble and of large molecular weight, parenchymal drug delivery is limited (Table 3). Consequently, the optimal treatment for systemic disease often does not cross the BBB. As a result, optimal treatment for BM is often different than that used to treat systemic disease. The BBB normally is a barrier to xenobiotic brain entrance however it is disrupted in patients with BM as evidenced by radiographic contrast enhancement. Consequently, the BM is permeable to chemotherapy agents that otherwise would not penetrate the BBB. However, brain adjacent to tumor (usually contaminated with tumor) and micrometastases within brain (tumors 1–3 millimeters in size) maintain an intact BBB and therefore are regions physically inaccessible to non-lipophilic and large molecular weight chemotherapy. Furthermore, the concomitant use of corticosteroids (most often dexamethasone) in patients with BM re-establishes the BBB and thereby limits chemotherapy access into brain/tumor. Lastly, up to 40% of patients with BM develop tumor-related seizures and accordingly are treated with hepatic cytochrome P450 inducing anticonvulsant drugs that alter the metabolism of a number of systemic chemotherapies. Several generalizations can be made regarding chemotherapy of BM based on the

Table 2. Outcome measures in brain metastases

- Survival
  - ➢ Overall
  - ➢ 6-month
  - ➢ 12-month
  - ➢ Brain-specific
- Time to tumor progression
- Control rate
  - ➢ Local
  - ➢ Distant
- Response rate
- Functional status
  - ➢ Karnofsky performance status
  - ➢ FACT-Brain

Table 3. Chemotherapy and BBB Passage [8]

Very good	Good	Poor	No penetration
ACNU	DTIC	VP-16	Taxanes
BCNU	MTX	Cisplatin	Gemcitabine
CCNU	Temozolomide	Carboplatin	CPT-11
Procarbazine	Ara-C	Vincristine	Cytokines
Hydroxyurea			
Topotecan			

limited literature. Response to chemotherapy reflects inherent chemosensitivity of the primary tumor with best responses seen with small cell lung cancer (SCLC), intermediate responses seen with non-small cell lung cancer (NSCLC) and low response rates with melanoma. Response to chemotherapy is in addition determined by prior chemotherapy exposure, as front-line chemotherapy has higher response rates than second- or third-line chemotherapy. Response to chemotherapy as compared to WBI or stereotactic radiotherapy is inferior and less durable in patients with SCLC, NSCLC and melanoma. The use of chemotherapy for the treatment of BM is most often limited to patients having failed radiotherapy (often both whole brain and stereotactic), with multiple lesions and in selected instances (for example solitary BM), surgical resection. The majority of chemotherapy trials for BM have utilized either single agent for example temozolomide or histology-specific multiagent chemotherapy. A less common chemotherapy approach has been the placement of carmustine wafers (Gliadel) in the bed of a resected and most often solitary metastasis. More recently, targeted therapies for example tyrosine kinase inhibitors such as erlotinib (Tarceva) and gefitinib (Iressa) have been used in patients with NSCLC and BM. These varying approaches are discussed in the subsequent sections.

Chemotherapy

Single Agent Chemotherapy

Temozolomide (TMZ) has been the chemotherapy agent studied most and not surprisingly, used most often in patients with refractory BM (Table 4) [9–15]. TMZ crosses the BBB (approximate serum to CSF ratio 0.33), has a favorable toxicity profile and has emerged as the chemotherapy agent of first choice for patients with gliomas. However, the data regarding efficacy in extraneural tumors is quite limited aside from melanoma and consequently TMZ is rarely used as a primary therapy for lung cancer. Several TMZ drug schedules have been used to treat BM (42/56; 75mg/m^2/day for 42 days with 14 day break in therapy: 21/28; 75–100mg/m^2/day for 21 days with 7 day break: and 5/28; 150–200mg/m^2/day for

Table 4. Single agent temozolomide for brain metastases

Author, year	Number of patients (primary)	Time to tumor progression (months)	Response (%)		
			Complete	Partial	Stable
Abrey[9]	41 (various)	2	0	5	37
Agarwala[10]*	117 (melanoma)	1	1	5	29
Christodoulou[11]	27 (various)	3	0	4	17
Dzidziuszko[12]	25 (NSCLC)	Not reported	0	0	25
Friedman[13]	52 (various)	Not reported	0	6	63
Giannitto[14]	9 (NSCLC)	Not reported	3	0	3
Siena[15]*	21 (NSCLC)	Not reported	0	8	24
	21 (melanoma)	Not reported	0	8	40
Schadendorf [48]*	45(melanoma)	<2 months	0	4.4	11.1
Boogerd [49]	52(melanoma)	7 months	6	4	12

*: no prior radiotherapy, TMZ used as first-line therapy

5 days with a 23 day break) though most commonly the 5/28 schedule has been utilized. As can be seen in Table 4, TMZ for BM results in neuroradiographic responses in approximately 5% (all partial responses) and 25% disease stabilization. However, median time to tumor progression is only 1 to 3 months. All but the trials by Sienna and Argawala administered TMZ as salvage therapy after evidence of disease progression following WBI. In the trial by Schadendorf et al a dose intensive TMZ schedule (7/14) was utilized for asymptomatic melanoma BM without prior application of WBI [48]. Response rate was 4% and median survival was 4 months. The best response data regarding single agent TMZ (5/28 schedule) was reported by Boogerd et al [49]. Amongst 52 patients (29 treated with TMZ only; 23 with TMZ and immunotherapy) with melanoma and small mostly asymptomatic (73%) BM, there were 5 responders (11%) with a median duration of response (including stable disease) of 7 months. These data suggest that TMZ has limited efficacy as a single agent in patients with BM though may provide palliation for a brief period of time.

Single agent fotemustine, a nitrosourea available in Europe, results in similar response rates and duration of response as TMZ in patients with melanoma and BM. In a trial by Jacquillat of 153 patients with metastatic melanoma of whom 36 (23%) had BM, fotemustine resulted in a 25% partial response rate with a median duration of response of 4 months [16].

Single agent topotecan (Table 5) has been investigated in several studies for the treatment of BM primarily due to its well-established activity and the fact that it freely penetrates the blood-brain barrier [50]. Lorusso et al. report on 19 patients with a variety of systemic cancers and BM treated with topotecan ($1.5mg/m^2$/day for 5-consecutive days every 3-weeks) [51]. Two responses were seen (both small cell lung cancer) however the trial was stopped for failing to meet pre-specified

Table 5. Single agent topotecan for brain metastases 50

Author, year	Number of patients (primary)	Time to tumor progression (months)	Response (%)		
			Complete	Partial	Stable
Larruso[51]	19 (various)	2	0	5	37
Oberhoff [52]	16 (breast)	Not reported	6	31	31
Manegold [53]*	16 (SCLC)	Not reported	25	38	31
Ardizzoni [54]	7 (SCLC)	1	43	14	0
Depierre[55]	9 (SCLC)	Not reported	11	44	33
Schutte[56]	24 (2 NSCLC; 22 SCLC)	Not reported	17	33	25
Korfel [57]	30 (SCLC)	Not reported	10	23	27

*: no prior radiotherapy, TMZ used as first-line therapy

efficacy criteria. In a phase 2 study of 92 patients with SCLC treated with topotecan (same schedule as above) and 7 patients with BM, Ardizzoni et al. reported that 3 patients achieved a complete response and one a partial response [54]. Similar response data is seen in Table 5 suggesting that topotecan is an active agent in patients with either breast cancer or small cell lung cancer.

Experience with targeted agents in the treatment of BM is limited and best characterized in NSCLC treated with gefitinib or erlotinib (Table 6)[17–21]. Intracranial response is predominantly seen in patients with responding concurrent systemic disease (usually Asian female nonsmokers with adenocarcinoma) and manifesting treatment- related rash.

Multiagent Chemotherapy

A number of nonrandomized trials have evaluated combination chemotherapy in patients with BM (Table 7) [22–35]. Notwithstanding higher response rates in SCLC, median survival is similar when comparing NSCLC to SCLC (approximately

Table 6. Epidermal growth factor receptor inhibitors as single agent therapy for NSCLC brain metastases

Author, year	Number of patients	Concurrent WBI	Intracranial response (%)			Median survival (months)
			Complete	Partial	Stable	
Cappuzzo[17]	4	3	25	75	0	6
Ceresoli[18]	41	18	0	10	17	3
Hotta[19]	14	0	7	36	57	9
Namba[20]	15	1	7	53	13	8.3
Shimato[21]	8	8	0	37.5	0	9.5

Table 7. Combination chemotherapy for brain metastases

Treatment (author)	Number of patients	Intracranial response (%)			Median survival (months)
		Complete	Partial	Stable	
NSCLC					
Carboplatin + VP-16 (Malacarne[22])	18	0	17	17	7.5
TPDCFH (Kaba[31])	39	3	10	13	6
Cisplatin + Vinorelbine (Robinet[23])	86	1	26	27	6
SCLC					
Carboplatin + VP-16 (Malacarne[22])	12	25	33	58	5.8
TPDCFH (Kaba[24])	9	33	33	66	8
Cytoxan + VP-16 + Adriamycin (Seute[25])	24	8	12.5	4	8.3
Cytoxan + VP-16 + Vincristine (Twelves[26])	14	7	57	Not reported	Not reported
VP-16 + Cytoxan + Doxorubicin + Vincristine (Lee[27])	11	9	13	Not reported	Not reported
VP-16 or VM-26 (Kristensen[28])	35	14	26		6
Cisplatin + Teniposide (Minotti[29])	23	13	22	Not reported	5
Melanoma					
TPDCFH (Kaba[31])	9	0	0	0	3
Temodar + Docetaxel (Bafaloukos[31])	8	0	38	38	3.5
Temodar + Carboplatin (Strauss[32])	11	0	0	0	Not reported
Temodar + Thalidomide (Hwu[33])	15	6.7	13	47	6
IL-2 + α-interferon + cisplatin + carmustine + dacarbazine (Richards[30])	15	0	47	0	6.5
Various					
Temodar + topotecan (Eckart [58])	25	0	12	28	Not reported
Temodar + vinorelbine (Omura [59])	18	0	6	39	Not reported
Temodar + cisplatin (Christopoulos [60])	32	3	28	16	2.9

TPDCFH: 6-thioguanine, procarbazine, dibromodulcitol, lomustine, 5-FU, hydroxyurea

Table 8. Pre-radiation chemotherapy for patients with brain metastases

Author, year	Number of patients	Chemotherapy	Response (%)			Duration of response (months)	Median survival (months)
			Complete	Partial	Stable		
NSCLC							
Fujita[34]	30	Cisplatin + Ifosfamide + CPT-11	0	12	11	5	13
Robinet[23]	60	Cisplatin + Navelbine	1	26			6
Franciosi[35]	43	Cisplatin + VP-16	7	23	35	8	8
Bernardo[36]	20	Gemcitabine + Navelbine + Carboplatin	15	30		6	7.5
Cortes[37]	26	Taxol + Gemsar	0	38		4	5
Moscetti[61]	110	Platinum couplet	27% (CR+PR)			6	11
SCLC							
Postmus[38]	60	Tenoposide	8	13	22	3.2	

Table 9. TMZ and WBI for brain metastases

Author	Number of patients	Response	Outcome
Antonadou[39]			No difference in median overall survival (8.6 vs. 7.0 months)
TMZ+WBI	25	96%	
WBI	23	67%	
Verger[40]			No difference in median overall survival (4.1 months)
TMZ+WBI	44	PFS-3: 72%	
WBI	41	PFS-3: 54%	
Margolin[41]	31 (melanoma)	10%	Not reported
Hofman[42]	34 (melanoma)	9%	7 month median survival

WBI: WBI
PFS-3: progression free survival at 3-months

7 months). In a recent study of SCLC and BM, Seute evaluated 181 consecutive patients with newly diagnosed SCLC by cranial MRI [25]. Twenty-four (13%) had asymptomatic BM compared to 38 patients (21%) with symptomatic BM. All patients were treated in a similar manner with respect to systemic chemotherapy (cytoxan, etoposide and doxorubicin). In patients with asymptomatic BM, the intracranial response rate was one third that of the systemic response rate (27% vs. 73%) suggesting that poor brain drug delivery limits response of BM to active systemic therapy. These results are similar to those reported by Kristensen in a review of BM response to chemotherapy in patients with SCLC (overall response 40%, Table 7)[29].

Multiagent therapy when compared to single agent TMZ appears to offer no advantage with respect to response rates in the treatment of BM and melanoma. Furthermore, duration of response to TMZ plus therapy and melanoma BM is limited to 3+ months in patients previously treated with systemic chemotherapy.

Pre-Radiation Chemotherapy

Several trials demonstrate the feasibility and safety of concurrent therapy in the treatment of patients with BM (Table 8)[23,36–40]. Robinet conducted a randomized trial in 171 patients with newly diagnosed BM and NSCLC. Patients received either upfront whole brain irradiation (WBI) or deferred radiotherapy at time of intracranial disease progression [23]. Both groups were treated with systemic cisplatin and navelbine chemotherapy. Response rates (both intracranial and extracranial), progression free survival and overall survival were similar in both groups. Two thirds of patients in the deferred radiotherapy group required radiotherapy. This trial suggests that in patients with NSCLC and synchronous BM, primary chemotherapy is a reasonable approach however patients require careful neurological follow-up. A similar finding (primary chemotherapy in patients with NSCLC and synchronous asyptomatic BM) was demonstrated in the survey evaluation by Christopoulos [61]. The Robinet trial of NSCLC is to be contrasted with that of Seute in patients with SCLC mentioned above wherein the intracranial response rate was one third that of the systemic disease response to chemotherapy. [26] Consequently, a majority of patients with BM required WBI. These studies suggest a subset of patients with either SCLC or NSCLC-related BM may respond to systemic chemotherapy permitting deferred radiotherapy.

Concurrent Chemotherapy and Radiotherapy

Antonadou studied 52 patients with BM and solid tumors (40 with lung cancer; 5 with breast cancer) in which patients were randomized to either WBI with or without TMZ. [41] The radiographic response rate was 96% (38% complete; 58% partial) in the TMZ arm compared to 67% (33% complete; partial 33%) in the radiotherapy only arm (p=0.017) [Table 9]. Margolin, in a single arm study of 31 patients with BM secondary to melanoma, treated with TMZ and WBI demonstrated a very modest response rate (1/31 complete; 2/31 partial). [43] In a similar study, Hofman treated

Table 10. Carmustine wafer implants in patients with brain metastases

	Ewend[43]	Golden[44]	Brem[45]
Number of patients	25	36	43
Local recurrence	0	0	1
Distant recurrence	4/25	7/36	2/43
Median survival	14.2 months	Not reported	17 months

34 patients with melanoma and BM with WBI and TMZ. [44] Observed response rate was 9% (3% complete; 6% partial) with a median progression free survival of 5 months and overall survival of 7 months. Ulrich treated 12 patients with metastatic melanoma and BM with WBI and concurrent fotemustine. [45] A 50% response (33% complete; 17% partial) and 8 month median survival was reported. Two other studies, both in patients with NSCLC, utilized either daily topotecan (n=80) or once weekly placlitaxel (n=86) in conjunction with WBI reported a 10–12% response rate (all partial) and a median survival of 5–6 months.

Several novel strategies have been used to improve drug delivery to brain in patients with symptomatic BM. One strategy is by local administration using carmustine impregnated biodegradable wafers (Gliadel) [Table 10]. [22–48] This therapy is performed in patients undergoing surgical resection at which time Gliadel is implanted following which patients are treated with WBI. This therapy however is for select patients (surgical candidates, solitary metastasis in whom local control is paramount) and purportedly results in improved local control rates. Problematic with interpreting these studies is WBI is variously applied, metastatic tumors are treated either at presentation or recurrence and administration of systemic chemotherapy is usually not reported. Another strategy though less often used approach entails administration of intra-arterial chemotherapy with or without osmotic BBB disruption. Again this therapy is for select patients and can be performed only by centers skilled at intracerebral intra-arterial drug adminis-tration. [49] At present, it is unclear as to whether intra-arterial therapy is superior to alternative approaches discussed above and furthermore has associated risks as seen with invasive intra-arterial therapies. In aggregate, these studies suggest that chemotherapy and WBI may be synergistic in the treatment of BM and thereby result in improved radiographic responses. However less clear is whether there is benefit with respect to either neurological function or quality of life and brain-specific survival.

Conclusions

Chemotherapy has a limited role in the management of patients with BM secondary to lung cancer or metastatic melanoma. For the majority of patients with BM, primary therapy of symptomatic BM will be WBI except in patients with either solitary or oligometastatic disease. Surgery is of benefit in good risk patients i.e. RTOG RPA class1 and some class 2 and in patients with solitary BM. Whether added benefit in such good risk patients is achieved by placement of carmustine wafer implants at time of surgery is unclear. Furthermore, whether the use of Gliadel in patients with resected solitary BM can permit deferral of WBI is unknown. In patients with asymptomatic BM, primary chemotherapy and deferred WBI is reasonable however careful assessment of intracranial response is required. Often, the intracranial response is discordant with and less than the chemotherapy response of systemic disease. In this circumstance in which no response of BM to primary chemotherapy is seen, WBI would be administered. As the majority of patients with BM are treated with WBI, the question of whether concurrent chemotherapy adds benefit remains uncertain. A synergetic effect may be seen with respect to intracranial response though less certain is whether meaningful benefit is realized as overall survival appears similar in patients treated with or without chemotherapy and WBI. The major utility of systemic chemotherapy in the treatment of BM is in patients' refractory to radiotherapy and in which no other treatment options remain. In this limited context, chemotherapy may offer limited benefit though whether an advantage is seen with single versus multiagent chemotherapy is uncertain. The utility of targeted therapy and in particular small molecule inhibitors continues to evolve in oncology and hopefully will offer new therapies for patients with BM.

References

1. Buckner JC. The role of chemotherapy in the treatment of patients with brain metastases from solid tumors. Cancer Metastis Rev 1991; 10: 335–41.
2. Peereboom DM. Chemotherapy in Brain Metastases. Supplement to Neurosurgery 2005; 57: 54–65.
3. Lesser GJ. Chemotherapy of Cerebral Metastases from Solid Tumors. Neurosurgery Clinics of North America 1996; 7: 527–536.
4. Mehta MP, Khuntia, D. Current Strategies in Whole-Brain Radiation Therapy for Brain Metastases. Supplement to Neurosurgery 2005; 57: 33–44.
5. Greig NH. Chemotherapy of Brain Metastases: Current Status. Cancer Treatment Reviews 1984; 11: 157–186.
6. Langer CJ, Mehta MP. Current management of Brain Metastases, With a Focus on Systemic Options. Journal of Clinical Oncology 2005; 23: 6207–6219.
7. Gaspar L, Scott C, Rotman M, Asbell S, Phillips T, Wasserman T, McKenna WG, Byhardt R: Recursive partitioning analysis (RPA) of prognostic factors in three Radiation Therapy Oncology Group (RTOG) brain metastases trials. Int J Radiat Oncol Biol Phys 1997; 37:745–751.
8. Kortmann RD, Jeremic B, Weller M, Plasswilm L, Bamberg M. Radiochemotherapy of malignant glioma in adults: Clinical experiences. Strahlenther Onkol 2003; 179:219–232.

9. Abrey LE, Olson JD, Raizer JJ, Mack M, Rodavitch A, Boutros DY, Malkin MG: A phase II trial of temozolomide for patients with recurrent or progressive brain metastases. J Neuro-Oncology 2001; 53:259–265.

10. Agarwala SS, Kirkwood JM, Gore M, Dreno B, Thatcher N, Czarnetski B, Atkins M, Buzaid A, Skarlos D, Rankin EM. Temozolomide for the Treatment of Brain Metastases Associated with Metastatic Melanoma: A Phase II Study. Journal of Clin Oncol 2004; 22: 2101–2107.

11. Christodoulou C, Bafaloukos D, Kosmidis P, Samantas E, Bamias A, Papakostas P, Karabelis A, Bacoyiannis C, Skarlos DV: Phase II study of temozolomide in heavily pretreated cancer patients with brain metastases. Ann Oncol 2001; 12:249–254.

12. Dziadziuszko R, Ardizzoni A, Postmus PE, Smit EF, Price A, Debruyne C, Legrand C, Giaccone G. Temozolomide in patients with advanced non-small cell lung cancer with and without brain metastases: A phase II study of the EORTC Lung Cancer Group (08965). Eur J Cancer 2003; 39: 1271–1276.

13. Friedman HS, Evans B, Reardon D, Quinn J, Rich J, Gururangan S, Stafford-Fox V, Chen C, Pati A, Schmidt W: Phase II trial of temozolomide for patients with progressive brain metastases. Proc Am Soc Clin Oncol 2003; 22: 102 (abstr).

14. Giannitto-Giorgio C, Cordio S, Di Blasi C. Temozolomide shows promising activity against pretreated brain recurrences of NSCLC. Preliminary results of a phase II trial (abstr). Proc Am Soc Clin Oncol 2002; 21 (abstr).

15. Siena S, Landonio G, Baietta E, Vitali M, Crinò L, Danova M, Musolino A, Gardin G, Foa P, Fincato G. Multicenter phase II study of temozolomide therapy for brain metastasis in patients with malignant melanoma, breast cancer, and non-small cell lung cancer. Proc Am Soc Clin Oncol 2003; 22:102 (abstr).

16. Jacquillat C, Khayat D, Banzet P, Weil M, Fumoleau P, Avril MF, Namer M, Bonneterre J, Kerbrat P, Bonerandi JJ, Bugat R, Monteuquet P, Cupissol D, Lauvin R, Vilmer C, Prache C, Bizzari JP. Final Report of the French Multi-center Phase II Study of the Nitrosourea Fotemustine in 153 Evaluable Patients with Disseminated Malignant Melanoma including Patients with Cerebral Metastases. Cancer 1990; 66: 1873–1878.

17. Cappuzzo F, Ardizzoni A, Soto-Parra H, Gridelli C, Maione P, Tiseo M, Calandri C, Bartolini S, Santoro A, Crino L. Epidermal Growth Factor Receptor Targeted Therapy by ZD 1839 (Iressa) in Patients with Brain Metastases from Non-Small Cell Lung Cancer (NSCLC). Lung Cancer 2003; 41: 227–231.

18. Ceresoli GL, Cappuzzo F, Gregorc V, Bartolini S, Crinó L, Villa E. Gefitinib in Patients with Brain Metastases from Non-Small-Cell Lung Cancer: a Prospective Trial. Annals of Oncology 2004; 15: 1042–1047.

19. Hotta K, Kiura K, Ueoka H, Tabata M, Fujiwara K, Kozuki T, Okada T, Hisamoto A, Tanimoto M. Effect of Gefitinib ('Iressa', ZD1839) on Brain Metastases in patients with advanced non-small cell lung cancer. Lung Cancer 2004; 46: 255–261.

20. Namba Y, Kijima T, Yokota S, Niinaka M, Kawamura S, Iwasaki T, Yoshito T, Kimur s in Patients with Advanced Non-Small-Cell Lung Cancer. Lung Cancer 2004a H, Okada T, Yamaguchi T, Nakagawa M, Okumura Y, Maeda H, Ito M. Gefitinib in Patients with Brain Metastases from Non-Small-Cell Lung Cancer: Review of 15 Clinical Cases. Clinical Lung Cancer 2004; 6: 123–128.

21. Shimato S, Mitsudomi T, Kosaka T, Yatabe Y, Wakabayashi T, Mizuno M, Nakahara N, Hatano H, Natsume A, Ishii D, Yoshida J. EGFR Mutations in Patients with Brain Metastases from Lung Cancer: Association with the Efficacy of Gefitinib. Neuro-Oncology 2006; 8: 137–144.

22. Malacarne P, Santini A, Maestri A. Response of Brain metastases from lung cancer to systemic chemotherapy with carboplatin and etoposide. Oncology 1996; 53:210–213.

23. Robinet G, Thomas P, Breton JL, Lena H, Gouva S, Dabouis G, Bennouna J, Souquet PJ, Balmes P, Thiberville L, Fournel P, Quoix E, Riou R, Rebattu P, Perol M, Paillotin D, Mornex F: Results of a phase III study of early versus delayed whole brain radiotherapy with concurrent cisplatin and vinorelbine combination in inoperable brain metastasis of non-small-cell lung cancer: Groupe Francais de Pneumo-Cancerologie (GFPC) Protocol 95–1. Ann Oncol 2001; 12:59–67.

24. Kaba SE, Kyritsis AP, Hess K, Yung WK, Mercier R, Dakhill S, Jaeckle KA, Levin VA: TPDC-FuHu chemotherapy for the treatment of recurrent metastatic brain tumors. J Clin Oncol 1997; 15:1063–1070.

25. Seute T, Leffers P, Wilmink JT, ten Velde Guul PM, Twijnstra A. Response of Asymptomatic Brain Metastases from Small-Cell Lung Cancer to Systemic First-Line Chemotherapy. Journal of Clinical Oncology 2006; 24 2079—2083.

26. Twelves CJ, Souhami RL, Harper PG, et al: The response of cerebral metastases in small cell lung cancer to systemic chemotherapy. Br J Cancer 1990; 61: 147–150.

27. Lee JS, Murphy WK, Glisson BS, et al: Primary chemotherapy of brain metastasis in small-cell lung cancer. J Clin Oncol 7:916–922, 1989.

28. Kristensen CA, Kristjansen PEG, Hansen HH. Systemic Chemotherapy of Brain Metastases from Small-Cell Lung Cancer: A Review. Journal of Clinical Oncology 1992; 10, 1498–1502.27.

29. 29. Minotti V, Crino L, Meacci ML, Corgna E, Darwish S, Palladino MA, Betti M, Tonato M. Chemotherapy with Cisplatin and Teniposide for Cerebral Metastases in Non-Small Cell Lung Cancer. Lung Cancer 1998; 20: 93–98.

30. Richards JM, Gale D, Mehta N, Lestingi T. Combination of Chemotherapy with Interleukin-2 and Interferon Alfa for the Treatment of Metastatic Melanoma. Journal of Clinical Oncology 1999; 17, 651–660.

31. Bafaloukos D, Gogas H, Georgoulias V, Briassoulis E, Fountzilas G, Samantas E, Kalofonos CH, Temozolomide in Combination with Docetaxel in Patients with Advance Melanoma: A Phase II Study of the Hellenic Cooperative Oncology Group. Journal of Clinical Oncology 2002; 20: 420–425.

32. Strauss SJ, Marples M, Napier MP, Meyer T, Boxall J, Rustin GJ: A phase I (tumour site-specific) study of carboplatin and temozolomide in patients with advanced melanoma. B J Cancer 2003; 89: 1901–1905.
33. Hwu W, Lis E, Menell JH, Panageas KS, Lamb LA, Merrell J, Williams LJ, Krown SE, Chapman PB, Livingston PO, Wolchok JD, Houghton AN. Temozolomide plus Thalidomide in Patients with Brain Metastases from Melanoma. Cancer 2005; 103:2590–2597.
34. Fujita A, Fukuoka S, Takabatake H, Tagaki S, Sekine K: Combination chemotherapy of cispllatin, ifosfamide, and irinotecan with rhG-CSF support in patients with brain metastases from non-small cell lung cancer. Oncology 2000; 59:291–295.
35. Franciosi V, Cocconi G, Michiara M, Di Costanzo F, Fosser V, Tonato M, Carlini P, Boni C, Di Sarra S. Front-Line Chemotherapy with Cisplatin and Etoposide for Patients with Brain Metastases from Breast Carcinoma, Nonsmall Cell Lung Carcinoma, or Malignant Melanoma. American Cancer Society 1999; 85, 1599–1605.
36. Bernardo G, Cuzzoni Q, Strada MR, Bernardo A, Brunetti G, Jedrychowska I, Pozzi, U, Palumbo R. First-Line Chemotherapy with Vinorelbine, Gemcitabine, and Carboplatin in the Treatment of Brain Metastases from Non-Small-Cell Lung Cancer: A Phase II Study. Cancer Investigation 2002; 20, 293–302.
37. Cortes J, Rodriguez J, Aramendia JM, Salgado E, Gurpide A, Garcia-Foncillas J, Aristu JJ, Claver A, Bosch A, Lopez-Picazo JM, Martin-Algarra S, Brugarolas A, Calvo E. Front-Line Paclitaxel/Cisplatin-Based Chemotherapy in Brain Metastases from Non-Small-Cell Lung Cancer. Oncology 2003; 64:28–35.
38. Postmus PE, Haaxmo-Reiche H, Smit EF, Groen HJM, Karnicka H, Lewinski T, Meerbeeck JV, Clerico M, Gregor A, Curran D, Sahmoud T, Kirkpatrick A, Gioccone G. Treatment of Brain Metastases of Small-Cell Lung Cancer: Comparing Teniposide and Teniposide with Whole-Brain Radiotherapy-A Phase III Study of the European Organization for the Research and Treatment of Cancer Lung Cancer Cooperative Group. J Clin Oncol 2000; 18:3400–3408.
39. 39. Antonadou D, Paraskevaidis M, Sarris G, Coliarakis N, Economou I, Karageorgis P, Throuvalas N. Phase II Randomized Trial of Temozolomide and Concurrent Radiotherapy in Patients with Brain Metastases. J Clin Oncol 2002; 20: 3644–3650.
40. 40.Verger E, Gil M, Yaya R, Vinolas N, Villa S, Pujol T, Quinto L, BSc, Graus F. Temozolomide and Concomitant Whole Brain Radiotherapy in Patients with Brain Metastases: A Phase II Randomized Trial. Internat J Radiat Oncol Bio Phy 2005; 61:185–191.
41. Margolin K, Atkins B, Thompson A, Ernstoff S, Weber J, Flaherty L, Clark I, Weiss G, Sosman J, Smith W, Dutcher P, Gollob J, Longmate J, Johnson D. Temozolomide and whole brain irradiation in melanoma metastatic to the brain: A phase II trial of the Cytokine Working Group. J Clin Oncol 2002; 128:214–218.

42. Hofman M, Kiecker F, Wurm R, Schlenger L, Budach V, Sterry W, T Uwe. Temozolomide with or without radiotherapy in melanoma with unresectable brain metastases. Journal of Neuro-Oncology 2006; 76(1); 59–64.

43. Ulrich J, Gademann G, Gollnick H. Management of Cerebral Metastases from Malignant Melanoma: Results of a Combined, Simultaneous Treatment with Fotemustine and Irradiation. Journal of Neuro-Oncology 1999; 43: 173–178.

44. Ewend MG, Hobbs KB. Treatment of recurrent CNS metastases using BCNU-polymer wafers. Presented at the 72nd Annual Meeting of the American Association of Neurological Surgeons, Orlando, Florida, May 1–6, 2004 (abstr).

45. Golden GA, Meldorf M, PROLONG Study Group. Patients with metastatic brain cancer, undergoing resection and Gliadel implantation experienced low local recurrence rates in the PROLONG Registry. Presented at the annual meeting of the Society of Neuro-Oncology Toronto, ON, Canada, November 18–21, 2004 (abstr).

46. Brem S, Sampath R, Staller A, Panattil, Entis S, Chamberlain M. Local control of brain metastases after craniotomy, radiation therapy and implantable chemotherapeutic wafers. American Association of Neurological Surgeons. San Francisco, CA April 22–26, 2006. J Neurosurg 104(4):A698, 2006. (abstr)

47. Newton HB, Slivka MA, Volpi C, et al. Intra-arterial carboplatin and intravenous etoposide for treatment of metastatic brain tumors. J Neuro-Oncology 2003; 61: 35–44.

48. Schadendorf D, Hauschild A, Ugurel S, Thoelke A, Egberts F, Kreissig M, Linse R, Trefzer U, Vogt T, Tilgen W, Mohr P, garbe C. Dose-intensified biweekly Temozolomide in patients with asymptomatic brain metastases from malignant melanoma: a phase 2 DeCOG/ADO study. Ann Oncol 2006; 17 (10). 1592–7.

49. Boogerd W, de Gast GC, Dalesio O. Temozolomide in advanced malignant melanoma with small brain metastases: can we withhold cranial irradiation? Cancer 2007; 109: 306–12.

50. Wong E, Berkenblit A. The role of topotecan in the treatment of brain metastases. 2004. CME. TheOncologist.com.

51. Lorusso V, Galetta D, Giotta F, Rinaldi A, Romito S, Brunetti C, Silverstris N, Colucci G. Topotecan in the treatment of brain metastases:a phase 2 study of GOIM (Gruppo Oncologico dell'Italia Meridionale). Anticancer Res 2006; 26 (3B): 2259–63.

52. Oberoff C, Kieback DG, Wurstlein R, et al. Topotecan chemotherapy in patients with breast cancer and brain metastses: results of a pilot study. Onkologie 2001; 24: 256–260.

53. Manegold C, Pawel JV, Scheithauer W, et al. Response of SCLC brain metastases to toptotecan therapy. Ann Oncol 1996; 7 (suppl 50): 106–7.

54. Ardizzoni A, Hansen H, Dombernowsky P, et al. Topotecan, a new active drug in the second-line treatment of small cell lung cancer: a phase 2 study in patients with refractory and sensitive disease. J Clin Oncol 1997; 15: 2090–2096.

55. Depierre A, von Pawel J, Hans K, et al. Evaluation of topotecan (Hycamtin) in relapsed small cell lung cancer (SCLC).: a multicenter phase 2 study. Lung cancer 1997; 18 (suppl 1): 35.
56. Schutte W, Manegold C, von Pawel JV. Topotecan in the therapy of brain metastses in lung cancer. Onkologie 1998; 21 (suppl 4): 25–27.
57. Korfel A, Oehm C, von Pawel JV, et al. Response to topotecan of symptomatic brain metastses of small cell lung cancer after whole brain radiotherapy: a multicenter phase 2 study. Eur J Cancer 2002; 38: 1724–29.
58. Eckardt JR, Martin KA, Schmidt AM, et al. A phase 1 trial of intravenous topotecan in combination with oral Temozolomide daily times 5 every 28 days. Proc Am Soc Clin Oncol 2002: 21: 83b (abstract).
59. Omuro AM, raizer JJ, Demopoulos A, Malkin M, Abrey LE. Vinorelbine combined with a protracted course of temozolomide for recurrent brain metastases: a phase 1 trial. J Neurooncol 2006; 78 (3): 277–80.
60. Christodoulou C, Bafaloukos D, Linardou H, Aravantinos G, Bamias A, Carina M, Klouvas G, Skarlos D. Temozolomide combined with cisplatin in patients with brain metastses from solid tumors: a Hellenic Cooperative Oncology Group phase 2 study. J Neurooncol 2005; 71 (1): 61–5.
61. Moscetti L, Nelli F, Felici A, Rinaldi M, DeSantis S, D'Auria G, Mansueto G, Tonini G, Sperduti I, Pollera FC. Up-front chemotherapy and radiation treatment in newly diagnosed nonsmall cell lung cancer with brain metastases: survey by Outcome Research Network for Evaluation of Treatment Results in Oncology. Cancer 2006; 109 (2): 274–281.

12. Palliative Care for Patients With Brain Metastases

Keren Barfi, M.D., Herbert Newton M.D., FAAN, Jamie Von Roenn, M.D.

Keywords: palliative care, brain metastases, corticosteroids, venous thromboembolism, cancer-related fatigue, neurocognitive deficits

Introduction

Brain metastases are an increasingly common complication of systemic malignancies. Systemic therapies continue to improve however not all cross the blood brain barrier, making brain metastases a manifestation of cancer that more practitioners are likely to encounter. Once the development of brain metastases has occurred, prognosis remains poor and there is an inevitable need to deal with the medical complications and to palliate symptoms that are prevalent amongst these patients. This chapter aims to cover the immediate medical issues and the supportive care and end of life issues that providers will encounter in the patient with brain metastases. Complications such as cerebral edema, seizures, venous thromboembolism, fatigue as well as neurocognitive and physical impairment will be addressed, along with recommendations regarding their management. Diligent consideration need be given to the side effects of any therapy that is instituted with a strong focus on maintaining quality of life throughout therapy.

Medical Issues in Patients with Brain Metastases

Steroid Treatment

Upon diagnosis of brain metastases, initiation of steroids has become standard of care and is absolutely indicated in those patients with symptomatic peritumoral edema [1, 2, 3]. In those patients with radiographic evidence of peritumoral edema and no clinical symptoms, steroids are not definitively needed, however, they are often administered nonetheless [3]. The beneficial effect of steroids in this setting is derived from a reduction in vasogenic edema associated with the tumor mass itself; it is this vasogenic edema that is believed to be the cause of symptoms in this setting. Though the mechanism is not entirely understood, it is thought that corticosteroids stabilize an otherwise leaky blood brain barrier as well as reduce the permeability of tumor capillaries [3]. Once treatment is begun, resolution or improvement of symptoms occurs quickly, often within hours. Dexamethasone is the usual agent of choice because of its long half life and minimal mineralocorticoid activity [3]. Most patients are started on dexamethasone 16mg/day in divided doses. However, it must be stressed that any dosage of steroids is empirically chosen as there is no definitive data to clarify an optimal dose. In fact, some evidence suggests in cases of mild symptoms, lower doses are acceptable [4]. Vecht et al. studied the relationship between dexamethasone dosage and steroid side effects. This is one of the few studies of dosing and established that dexamethasone 4mg was often adequate to control patients' symptoms [4]. On the other hand, if symptoms persist or worsen, the dose may be increased. Dexamethasone has been used in doses as high as 100mg/day. Certainly, the minimal dosage necessary is recommended in order to avoid the many unwanted side effects of this class of drugs. Once a patient's symptoms have stabilized, steroids should be tapered to a minimally tolerated dose. The rate of steroid taper should be guided by the patient's response to changes in medication dosage. It is well known that some patients experience symptoms of "steroid withdrawal". These symptoms can include fatigue, somnolence, depressive symptoms and recrudescence of their neurological symptoms. In some cases, the doses may even need to be temporarily increased or maintained until a taper can be resumed. Occasionally patients may require long term use of steroids; in this case the goal would be once daily dosing.

Steroid Side Effects

Despite their clinical effectiveness, steroids can be associated with significant toxicity, both acutely and chronically (see Table 1). This can be difficult to manage in oncology patients who are often already very symptomatic from either their primary or metastatic disease. Of the many potential side effects, three are particularly important to consider in this patient population: Pneumocystis jirovecii pneumonia (PJP), steroid myopathy, and neurologic side effects.

Pneumocystis jirovecii Pneumonia

Pneumocystis jirovecii, previously known as Pneumocystis carinii, is a fungal infection capable of causing severe and potentially life threatening pneumonitis in immunocompromised patients. Though most commonly seen in patients with HIV/AIDS, solid organ transplant recipients and hematological malignancies, it is well documented that patients with solid tumors receiving corticosteroids are

Table 1. Corticosteroid Side Effects

Non Neurologic Mild Effects	Non Neurologic Serious Effects	Common Neurologic Effects	Uncommon Neurologic Effects
Weight gain	GI bleeding	Insomnia	Psychosis
Cushingoid features	Hyperglycemia/ Diabetes	Hiccups	Delirium
Candidiasis	Osteoporosis	Tremor	Seizures
Cataracts	Osteonecrosis (hip)	Visual blurring	
Dyspepsia	Opportunistic Infections	Behavioral changes	
Edema	Glaucoma	Myopathy	
Hirsuitism			
Acne			
Abdominal Bloating			

Adapted from El Kamar, F [1].

susceptible as well [5]. More specifically, it appears to be patients with primary brain tumors who are at highest risk. A retrospective study from Johns Hopkins Medical Institutions (JHMI) from 1980–2001, identified 110 cases of PCP amongst patients with an underlying malignancy. Of these 14% had primary brain tumors and 23% had other solid tumors, the remainder had hematological malignancies. Interestingly, the incidence of PCP infection amongst solid tumor patients had increased from 0% of all cases in 1980-1985 to 42% of all cases reported from 1996-2000 [5]. The authors noted that the use of steroids in this setting had not changed at the institution over that 20 year period. However the use of more aggressive and immunosuppressing therapies had increased. Therefore, they concluded that it was the combination of therapies in the treatment of brain tumors that was putting patients at increased risk of PCP infection.

Known risk factors for the development of PJP include: presence of lymphopenia, dosage and duration of treatment with corticosteroids. Many retrospective reviews have also identified that the period of highest risk for developing PJP occurs during steroid taper [6]. Though each of these studies is a small retrospective review, the outcomes appear to be consistent that patients with primary brain tumors have a substantial risk of developing this life-threatening infection.

Currently it is recommended that patients receiving a prolonged course of corticosteroids be given prophylaxis against PJP. Multiple options exist for prophylaxis including trimethoprim-sulfamethoxazole, dapsone, inhaled pentamidine or atovaquone. For the palliative care patient, the potential benefit of prophylactic medications needs to weighed against the goals of care which often include a minimization of pill burden and potential drug side-effects.

Steroid Myopathy

Prolonged use of high dose corticosteroids also predisposes patients to the development of steroid myopathy which is reported to occur in 20–60% of patients, though the true incidence is likely underestimated [7, 8]. The most susceptible patients are those who are elderly and on high dosages for a prolonged time course. Proximal muscle weakness is the defining feature and patients may complain of difficulty rising from a seated position, difficulty climbing stairs or fatigue with any lifting. Respiratory muscles can be affected as well leading to symptomatic dyspnea. Physical exam may be notable for weakness in the neck flexors and muscles of the shoulder and pelvic girdle. Studies evaluating the relationship between dexamethasone dosage and development of steroid myopathy have been performed. Vecht et al. performed a double-blind study evaluating the effect of dexamethasone dosage on Karnofsky performance status [4]. In this study 14% of patients on 4mg of dexamethasone developed proximal muscle weakness in comparison to 38% of patients on either 8mg or 16mg dexamethasone. Another study by Batchelor et al. prospectively evaluated fifteen adult cancer patients on steroid treatment to determine the frequency and time course of muscle weakness [8]. Notably, most patients became significantly weak within fifteen days of steroid treatment, thus challenging previous notions that myopathy can take several weeks or months to develop. Another important finding was that weakness in respiratory muscles, severe enough to cause dyspnea, could occur in the absence of proximal limb muscle weakness.

Steroid myopathy is an important cause of morbidity amongst patients with brain metastases. Because of its subacute onset and the potential for other concomitant focal neurological deficits in patients with brain metastases, physicians need to have a high index of suspicion in order to detect this debilitating condition early. Patients on corticosteroids should frequently have their proximal muscle strength tested at the bedside to monitor for any changes. Other more extensive evaluation to confirm the diagnosis is unnecessary because labs such as creatinine phosphokinase (CPK) or aldolase are usually normal and electromyogram (EMG) testing is most often unrevealing [3]. Once steroid myopathy develops, withdrawal of steroids and physical therapy are the only therapeutic options. If steroids must be continued, then the smallest possible dose should be used. After steroids are withdrawn, the muscle weakness is potentially completely reversible. Because the physical disabilities associated with brain metastases are often distressing to these patients, physicians should remain vigilant in evaluating for this iatrogenic cause of weakness and the secondary problem of deconditioning as well.

Central Nervous System (CNS) Side Effects

The use of systemic corticosteroids is well known to cause behavioral and mood changes, which can range from very mild to quite severe. Common CNS effects include mild mania, insomnia, hiccups, tremor and appetite stimulation. Most behavioral changes are likely to be mild however; the greater concern is the possible development of steroid psychosis. Data regarding this issue comes mostly in the form of case reports dating back to the early 1950's when corticosteroids were first introduced. The term steroid psychosis is apparently used indiscriminately in the literature and has been used inaccurately to describe any behavioral or psychic change occurring while on steroids, therefore estimating the true incidence of this complication remains challenging [9].

A recent review of the literature studied 130 cases of steroid psychosis reported between the years 1950–2002 [9]. It should be noted that this review was not intended to study patients with brain metastases. Two main profiles were proposed: affective and toxic-organic profile. The affective, refers to mania and depression which were significantly more common, accounting for 75% of reported cases, with mania being more common than depression within this category. The toxic-organic profile was defined by delirium and psychosis which occurred in 25% of reported cases. Early signs of the affective symptoms include: hyperactivity, euphoria, irritability or pressured speech. Early signs of the toxic-organic profile include: agitation, confusion, delusions and even hallucinations. The frequency of steroid psychosis is not well documented and potential risk factors are not well defined. There is some suggestion that women are more susceptible than men. However other factors such as advanced age or history of previous psychiatric illness have not been confirmed as predisposing factors. Onset of symptoms can be as early as four days after initiation of steroid therapy. Duration of symptoms varies according to the manifestation, with delirium resolving faster than either psychosis or mania.

As with all other serious corticosteroid side effects, treatment consists of medication withdrawal, along with use of a phenothiazine or other major tranquilizer. If steroids cannot be discontinued, one may continue steroids at the minimum dose required and add a neuroleptic medication. One case report noted improvement in 84% of patients who were treated in this fashion [10]. A few studies have shown that one episode of steroid psychosis does not predispose a patient to developing this complication again [10]. However clinical experience has also shown that some patients will unfortunately develop behavioral changes when retreated with steroids. Anecdotally, complete recovery was reported in more than 90% of cases. This is now being reconsidered as more recent studies have recognized long term complications such as memory impairment and possibly an increased risk of developing persistent symptoms of a bipolar disorder [10].

Other Side Effects to Consider

Patients being treated with corticosteroids are at risk for a multitude of side effects, some of the most serious of which were reviewed above. Other side effects that are often perceived as being distressing to patients include: cushingoid facies, hirsuitism, acne, reduced taste and abdominal bloating. From a provider's

primary caregiver present at home. The Medicare Benefit will continue to pay for patients who live longer than 6 months, as long as the attending physician continues to certify the patient is terminally ill. Most patients admitted to Hospice do not live longer than the typical 6 months allowed by the Medicare Benefit. In fact, the majority of them die within 4–6 weeks, suggesting that physicians are not referring their patients to Hospice care early enough [44]. Recent statistics show that more than one half of all terminally ill cancer patients in the United States are not being offered Hospice services at all or are entering Hospice care too late to achieve maximal benefit [43].

For MBT patients in whom continued treatment is futile, the most important and critical step will be to broach the subject of hospice care and palliative symptom control [46–48]. Similar to when the physician first tells the patient their diagnosis, this must be done with the utmost compassion and sensitivity. Patients should be referred to Hospice as soon as curative or stabilizing therapy has been discontinued and the primary goal becomes comfort. Hospice care works best when there is time for members of the Hospice team to develop meaningful relationships with the patient and family (i.e., over weeks to months).

The purpose of Hospice care is to provide medical, psychosocial, and spiritual support for terminally ill patients and their families [42–48]. This is an especially critical time when hope for cure is lost and anxiety about the future is overwhelming. Hospice care attempts to alleviate the physical and emotional suffering of the MBT patient. Hope for cure is shifted to hope for maximizing dignity, comfort, quality of life (QOL), and the process of enjoying each remaining day to its fullest. In addition, support is provided for the family members, who are also suffering and attempting to cope with the imminent loss of their loved on [49]. One of the most common fears about advanced incurable cancer is isolation from family and loved ones. The presence of the Hospice care team, especially in the home setting, alleviates this fear and ensures that isolation and loneliness are minimized.

The use of Hospice is an important aspect of the complete care of virtually all patients with neuro-oncologic disease. It should be offered to all patients in the terminal stages of their disease once efforts to halt the progression of the malignancy have ceased. In addition to expertise at treating many aspects of cancer-related pain, Hospice physicians and nurses can also effectively manage some of the problems specific to MBT patients, such as swallowing difficulties and seizures [50]. During the terminal phases of disease, many patients cannot take oral anticonvulsants properly, either due to neurological compromise of the swallowing mechanism or a reduced level of consciousness. It is often helpful for the Hospice nurse to administer these medications rectally as a suspension (using a dose that is approximately 25% higher than the oral dose). Sublingual valium drops can also be used, if needed, to augment seizure control. Patients with respiratory compromise and dyspnea may benefit from the use of opioids, with the dose depending on the level of prior exposure to this class of medications [51].

Ethical Issues

The care of neuro-oncology patients is often complicated by numerous ethical dilemmas and discussions [52–55]. In no other subspecialty of medicine are there such large numbers of seriously ill patients in which the day-to-day care involves life and death decisions. These patients are not only adversely affected by their disease, but frequently suffer deleterious side effects and complications from treatment, which is often very intense and rigorous. Physicians caring for MBT patients should be well versed in ethical principles and theory. This foundation will better prepare the physician for the many complex ethical predicaments that inevitably develop during the course of therapy and, in many cases, subsequent palliative care.

There are several basic ethical principles that require definition. The most important ethical principles are respect for autonomy, justice, beneficence, and non-maleficence [52–54]. *Respect for Autonomy* refers to recognition by the physician of the patient's right and ability to make his own decisions. These decisions are unique, are influenced by the patient's value system, and may differ from what is advised by the physician. *Justice* relates to fairness and what people are legitimately entitled to once they enter the medical system. In this context, justice demands that patients with MBT have access to care (e.g., treatment, pain control, nutritional support) equal to patients with other diseases that may have a less grave prognosis. *Beneficence* refers to actions by the physician towards the patient that will maximize positive outcomes and avoid unnecessary pain, injury, and suffering. These activities can include treatment of the cancer and extension of quality survival, control of pain and other disease-related symptoms, and interpersonal support. *Non-maleficence* means that the physician should "do no harm" while providing care to the patient. This principle has a broad scope and can refer to many issues, including withholding relevant diagnostic or prognostic information, improper treatment of pain, inappropriate under-treatment, and persistent over-treatment.

Physicians usually have an ethical position or frame of reference that incorporates these basic ethical principles. The most common ethical stance is that in which the physician makes a decision based on an assessment of the good or bad consequences of each course of action. This ethical position, called *consequentialism* or *utilitarianism*, justifies a given decision by comparing probable good or benefit with potential harm or pain [56]. The second most common ethical position, *respect for persons*, relies heavily on the ethical principles of autonomy and respect [52]. This approach emphasizes the importance of allowing patients to be involved in all decisions about their care and treatment. An alternative to *respect for persons* is *paternalism*, in which the physician assumes that all decisions should be made for the good of the patient, without regard to his or her specific wishes or needs [52–54,56].

It is often difficult to be honest with a patient when discussing a new diagnosis as devastating as cancer, especially when it is a MBT or similar neuro-oncologic problem [43–54,57,58]. In fact, a survey of ethical issues in the oncology literature determined that *truth-telling* was the most commonly debated subject [56]. Between

1961 and 1979, most physicians took the paternalistic approach and withheld information regarding diagnosis and prognosis in order to maintain hope and minimize psychological damage to their patients. Since 1979, attitudes have changed so that many physicians now prefer to reveal accurate information about their patient's diagnosis and prognosis [57–59]. This trend away from paternalism, towards a more "patient-oriented" or "respect for persons" approach when discussing diagnosis and prognosis, is important since the vast majority of patients want to know as much as possible about their disease, treatment options, and chances of survival [58].

The physician caring for a MBT patient needs to balance the ethically appropriate duty to convey accurate information about diagnosis and prognosis with the equally important responsibility to nurture and maintain hope. However, it is now clear that a more honest and accurate diagnostic interview does not remove hope and is more likely to strengthen the physician-patient relationship [58, 60]. The physician should explore what hope means to each patient, since it can represent many different things, some of which will be separate from the hope for cure or lengthy survival.

Ethical issues arise frequently during the design and administration of clinical trials for oncology patients. The moral cornerstone of any clinical trial is the concept and practice of valid informed consent [58]. Valid consent has three features: the provision of adequate information, the absence of coercion, and the competence of the patient. Adequate information must be provided about tests, procedures, and treatments inherent in any clinical trial. Significant risks and benefits, if any, must be outlined. All serious risks that are likely to occur should be included. Any risk of death beyond a trivial risk should also be included, because death is such a serious evil that the patient must be made aware of any chance that it may occur [61]. Rational alternative treatment to the clinical trial in question must be presented by the physician in an open, objective, and unbiased manner. Alternative treatments should include those offered at other medical centers. One of the duties of the physician is to inform the patient of the consequences and probable outcome with no treatment at all. The patient should know that the final decision concerning any clinical trial is his or hers alone to make. Competency, in this setting, implies that the patient understands the information provided during the consent process and appreciates that it applies to him/her at that particular point in time.

The protection of the patient's best interests falls squarely and heavily on the shoulders of the physician seeking participation in the clinical trial [55]. The physician must take into account the influence of personal beliefs, biases, and academic ambitions before embarking on such endeavors. The focus of the physician who designs and performs clinical trials must always be on the need for conclusive proof of efficacy. A study designed according to rigorous scientific and ethical criteria can accrue patients with confidence and good faith.

The decision to stop therapy is often very difficult for patients, family members, and the treatment team [52–54,62,63]. It signals the "beginning of the end," when all reasonable hope for cure or prolonged stabilization is gone and the patient's death is imminent. These decisions usually arise when the patient has just progressed through the latest protocol and has often suffered further neurological deterioration. In many cases, the neurological status is quite poor, to a degree that functional ambulation, cognition, and verbal interaction are severely compromised. Although there are often other treatment options that could be offered, the physician must state clearly and honestly that further therapy will not significantly affect outcome. In this situation, it is critical to weigh the adverse effects of further therapy on QOL against the potential benefits for improvement of QOL and prolongation of survival, which would be extremely limited. The physician must reassure the patient and family that the termination of active treatment does not mean the physician will abandon them. Even though the focus of subsequent care will shift to comfort, pain relief, and symptom control, the physician will remain actively involved in the patient's care. In addition to questions about the potential for extension of survival, many patients and family members want to know if further treatment might improve neurological function. In other words, could the patient's current neurological status be reversed somewhat to enhance QOL for the time they have left? Neurological function is rarely restored or improved at these late stages of disease; it would be optimistic even to expect further therapy to stabilize the patient's condition.

Because QOL is so subjective and the behavior of neuro-oncologic disease can be so variable, the proper time to stop treatment will differ from patient to patient. Some patients accustomed to a high level of function cannot tolerate living their life in a severely compromised fashion while suffering the rigors of treatment. For others, the alterations of function and lifestyle are more easily accepted, so that simple survival is adequate, with less regard for the quality of existence.

Is it ethically appropriate to terminate therapy? If the physician has explained the situation properly and is acting in accordance with the wishes of the patient or family, the decision would be consistent with the principles of respect for autonomy, beneficience, and non-maleficence [52–54,62–64]. The physician would be acting to allow a more dignified, peaceful death without the rigors of active therapy. Active treatment is terminated to "promote the good," which is to let the patient die on their own terms. It would be ethically improper and contrary to the principle of non-maleficence for the physician to coerce or force the patient into undergoing further therapy.

Conclusions

Care of the patient with brain metastases involves addressing both immediate medical complications as well as supportive care issues. Steroids are invariably used when the initial diagnosis is made to treat peritumoral edema and its associated symptoms. Every attempt should be made to use the lowest dose necessary so as to minimize steroid associated complications. Other complications such as seizures and VTE occur with significant frequency. In the event of seizures, AEDs are required, otherwise prophylaxis is not indicated. These medications have many potential side effects and drug-drug interactions that require monitoring. Regarding VTE, heparinoids or coumadin may be used, though the former may be preferred. Heparinoids may be more efficacious than coumadin, and dosing is often easier and more reliable. Cancer-related fatigue is a very common complication that is not unique to patients with brain metastases. Patients with this symptom require evaluation and treatment for the five most common causes of fatigue: anemia, hypothyroidism, depression, pain, emotional distress and sleep disturbances. Lastly, patients with brain metastases often suffer neurocognitive changes ranging from mild memory impairment to severe dementia, as well as physical disability. Some deficits are present at the time of presentation, while others become more severe as the disease progresses. Patients can attempt physical, occupational and speech therapy as is appropriate. In some instances, pharmacologic therapies with psychostimulants may be useful. Though treatment of both systemic malignancies as well as brain metastases continues to improve, this population continues to have a very poor prognosis with relatively short survival and any therapy should focus on maintaining quality of life above all else. Hospice utilization should be considered for all patients with brain metastases as the vast majority will die of their brain or systemic disease or both.

References

1. El Kamar F, Posner J. Brain metastases. Semin Neurol 2004; 24:347–362.
2. Koehler P. Use of corticosteroids in neuro-oncology. Anti-Cancer Drugs 1995; 6:19–33.
3. Wen P, Schiff D, Kesari S, et al. Medical management of patients with brain tumors. J Neurooncol 2006 Jun 29; [Epub ahead of print].
4. Vecht C, Hovestadt A, Verbiest H et al. Dose-effect relationship of dexamethasone on Karnofsky performance in metastatic brain tumors: A randomized study of doses of 4, 8, and 16 milligrams per day. Neurology 1994; 44:675–680.
5. Mahindra A, Grossman S. Pneumocystis carinii pneumonia in HIV negative patients with primary brain tumors. J Neurooncol 2003; 63:263–270.
6. Wen P, Marks P. Medical management of patients with brain tumors. Curr Opin Oncol 2002; 14:299–307.
7. Naim M, Reed A. Enzyme elevation in patients with juvenile dermatomyositis and steroid myopathy. J Rheumatol 2006; 33:1392–1394.
8. Batchelor T, Taylor L, Thaler H, et al. Steroid myopathy in cancer patients. Neurology 1997; 48: 1234–38.
9. Sirois F. Steroid psychosis: A review. Gen Hosp Psychiatry 2003; 25:27–33.
10. Lewis D, Smith R. Steroid-induced psychiatric syndromes. A report of 14 cases and a review of the literature. J Affect Disord 1983; 5:319–32.
11. Batchelor T, DeAngelis L. Medical management of cerebral metastases. Neurosur Clin 1996; 7:435–446.

12. Cohen N, Strauss G, Lew R et al. Should prophylactic anticonvulsants be administered to patients with newly diagnosed cerebral metastases? A retrospective analysis. J Clin Oncol 1988; 6:1621–1624.
13. Glantz M, Cole B, Friedberg M et al. A randomized, blinded, placebo-controlled trial of divalproex sodium prophylaxis in adults with newly-diagnosed brain tumors. Neurology 1996; 46:985–991.
14. Forsyth P, Weaver S, Fulton D et al. Prophylactic anticonvulsants in patients with brain tumor. Can J Neurol Sci 2003; 30:106–112.
15. Glantz M, Cole B, Forsyth P et al. Practice parameter: Anticonvulsant prophylaxis in patients with newly diagnosed brain tumors: Report of the quality standards subcommittee of the American Academy of Neurology. Neurology 2000; 54:1886–1893.
16. Schiff D, DeAngelis L. Therapy of venous thromboembolism in patients with brain metastases. Cancer1994; 73:493–498.
17. Hutten B, Prins M, Gent M et al. Incidence of recurrent thromboembolic and bleeding complications among patients with venous thromboembolism in relation to both malignancy and achieved international normalized ratio: a retrospective analysis. J Clin Oncol 2000; 18:3078–83.
18. Agnes Y,Lee M, Levine M et al. Low-molecular-weight heparin versus a coumarin for the prevention of recurrent venous thromboembolism in patients with cancer. NEJM 2003; 349:146–153.
19. Escalante CP. Treatment of cancer-related fatigue: an update. Support Care Cancer 2003; 11:79–83.
20. Prue G, Rankin J. Allen J et al. Cancer-related fatigue: A critical appraisal. Eur J Cancer 2006; 42: 846–863.
21. Osoba D, Aaronson N, Muller M et al. Effect of neurological dysfunction on health-related quality of life in patients with high-grade glioma. J Neurooncol 1997; 34:263–278.
22. Servaes P, van der Werf S, Prins J et al. Fatigue in disease-free cancer patients compared with fatigue in patients with chronic fatigue syndrome. Support Care Cancer 2001; 9:11–7.
23. Mock V, Atkinson A, Barsevick A et al. National Comprehensive Cancer Network (NCCN) practice guidelines for cancer-related fatigue. Oncology 2000; 14:151–161.
24. Taillibert S, Delattre JY. Palliative care in patients with brain metastases. Curr Opin Oncol 2005; 17:588–592.
25. Cella D. The Functional Assessment of Cancer Therapy-Anemia (FACT-An) Scale: a new tool for the assessment of outcomes in cancer anemia and fatigue. Semin Hematol 1997; 34(3 Suppl 2):13–19.
26. Cella D. Zagari M, Vandoros C et al. Epoetin alfa treatment results in clinically significant improvements in quality of life in anemic cancer patients when referenced to the general population. J Clin Oncol 2003; 21:366–373.

27. National Comprehensive Cancer Network (NCCN) practice guidelines for cancer- and treatment-related anemia.
28. Geiser F, Hahn C, Conrad R et al. Interaction of psychological factors and the effect of epoetin alfa treatment in cancer patients on hemoglobin and fatigue. Support Care Cancer 2006 Aug 25; [Epub ahead of print].
29. Tchekmedyian N, Kallich J, McDermott A et al. The relationship between psychologic distress and cancer-related fatigue. Cancer 2003; 98:198–203.
30. van Weert E, Hoekstra-Weebers J, Otter R et al. Cancer-related fatigue: predictors and effects of rehabilitation. The Oncologist 2006; 11:184–196.
31. Galvao D, Newton R. Review of exercise intervention studies in cancer patients. J Clin Oncol 2005; 23:899–909.
32. Dimeo F, Fetscher S, Lange W et al. Effects of aerobic exercise on the physical performance and incidence of treatment-related complications after high-dose chemotherapy. Blood 1997; 90:3390–3394.
33. Bruera E, Brenneis C, Chadwick S et al. Methylphenidate associated with narcotics for the treatment of cancer pain. Cancer Treat Rep 1987; 71:67–70.
34. Wilwerding M, Loprinzi C, Mailliard J et al. A randomized, cross-over evaluation of methylphenidate in cancer patients receiving strong narcotics. Support Care Cancer 1995; 3:135–138.
35. Bruera E, Driver L, Barnes E et al. Patient-controlled methylphenidate for the management of fatigue in patients with advanced cancer: A preliminary report. J Clin Oncol 2003; 21:4439–4443.
36. Bruera E, Valero V, Driver L et al. Patient-controlled methylphenidate for cancer fatigue: A double-blind, randomized, placebo-controlled trial. J Clin Oncol 2006; 24: 2073–2078.
37. Rozans M, Dreisbach A, Lertora J et al. Palliative uses of methylphenidate in patients with cancer: A review. J Clin Oncol 2002; 20:335–339.
38. Meyers C, Weitzner M, Valentine A et al. Methylphenidate therapy improves cognition, mood, and function of brain tumor patients. J Clin Oncol 1998; 16:2522–2527.
39. Archibald Y, Lunn D, Ruttan L et al. Cognitive functioning in long-term survivors of high-grade glioma. J Neurosurg 1994; 80:247–253.
40. Meyers C, Smith J, Bezjak A et al. Neurocognitive function and progression in patients with brain metastases treated with whole-brain radiation and motexafin gadolinium: results of a randomized phase III trial. J Clin Oncol 2004; 22: 157–165.
41. DeAngelis L, Delattre J, Posner J. Radiation-induced dementia in patients cured of brain metastases. Neurology 1989; 39:789–796.
42. Rhymes J. Hospice care in America. JAMA 1990; 264:369–372.
43. Kinzbrunner BM. Ethical dilemmas in hospice and palliative care. Support Care Cancer 1995; 3:28–36.
44. Von Gunten CF, Neely KJ, Martinez J. Hospice and palliative care: Program needs and academic issues. Oncol 1996; 10:1070–1074.

45. Finlay IG, Higginson IJ, Goodwin DM, et al. Palliative care in hospital, hospice, at home: results from a systematic review. Ann Oncol 2002; 13:257–264.
46. Baile WF, Glober GA, Lenzi R, Beale EA, Kudelka AP. Discussing disease progression and end-of-life decisions. Oncol 1999; 13:1021–1031.
47. von Gunten CF. Discussing hospice care. J Clin Oncol 2003; 21:31s–36s.
48. Kahn MJ, Lazarus CJ, Owens DP. Allowing patients to die: Practical, ethical, and religious concerns. J Clin Oncol 2003; 21:3000–3002.
49. Brenner PR. Managing patients and families at the ending of life: Hospice assumptions, structures, and practice in response to staff stress. Cancer Investig 1997; 15:257–264.
50. D'Olimpio J. Contemporary drug therapy in palliative care: New directions. Cancer Investig 2001; 19:413–423.
51. Thomas JR, Von Gunten CF. Treatment of dyspnea in cancer patients. Oncol 2002; 16:745–750.
52. Latimer E. Ethical challenges in cancer care. J Palliative Care 1992; 8:65–70.
53. Smith TJ, Bodurtha JN. Ethical considerations in oncology: Balancing the interests of patients, oncologists, and society. J Clin Oncol 1995; 13:2464–2470.
54. Newton HB, Malkin MG. Ethical issues in neuro-oncology. Sem Neurol 1997; 17:219–226.
55. Vick NA, Wilson CB. Total care of the patient with a brain tumor. With considerations of some ethical issues. Neurol Clin 1985; 3:705–710.
56. Vanderpool HY, Weiss GB. Ethics and cancer: A survey of the literature. South Med J 1987; 80:500–506.
57. Gert B, Culver CM. Moral theory in neurologic practice. Sem Neurol 1984; 4:9–14.
58. Butow PN, Kazemi JN, Beeney LJ, Griffin AM, Dunn SM, Tattersall MHN. When the diagnosis is cancer. Patient communication experiences and preferences. Cancer 1996; 77:2630–2637.
59. Gert B, Nelson WA, Culver CM. Moral theory and neurology. Neurol Clin 1989; 7:681–696.
60. Clayton JM, Butow PN, Arnold RM, Tattersall MHN. Fostering coping and nurturing hope when discussing the future with terminally ill cancer patients and their caregivers. Cancer 2005; 103:1965–1975.
61. Culver CM, Gert B. Basic ethical concepts in neurologic practice. Sem Neurol 1984; 4:1–8.
62. Thomasma DC. The ethics of caring for the older patient with cancer: Defining the issues. Oncol 1992; 6:124–130.
63. Nelson WA, Bernat JL. Decisions to withhold or terminate treatment. Neurol Clin 1989; 7:759–774.
64. Bernat JL, Goldstein ML, Viste KM. The neurologist and the dying patient. Neurol 1996; 46:598–599.

Subject Index

Acute Lymphoblastic Leukemia (ALL), 157, 169
Acute Myelogenous Leukemia (AML), 158–159
Acute toxicities, 94, 100
American Academy of Neurology (AAN), 85–86, 200
American Cancer Society (ACS), 3, 4
American Society of Therapeutic Radiation Oncology, 104
Angiogenesis, 13–14
Anticonvulsant therapy , 55–58
Antiepileptic drugs (AED), 55–58, 85–86
  use of, 220–221

Basic fibroblast growth factor (bFGF), 13
Batson's plexus, 119, 123
Bcl-2 expression, 186
1,3-Bis(2-Chloroethyl)-1-Nitrosourea (BCNU), 105
Blood Brain Barrier (BBB), 14–15, 33–34, 86, 106, 169, 170, 174, 177–178, 186
Blood-brain barrier disruption (BBBD), 177–178
Brachytherapy, 102
Brain metastases, epidemiology and pathophysiology of, 1–15
Brain metastases, surgery for
  advantages, 75–76
  AED and, 85–86
  anatomic considerations, 81–84
  DVT and, 86
  indications, 76
  locoregional therapy, 86–87
  multiple brain metastasis, 78–79
  recurrent intracranial metastatic disease, 79
  RPA classification, 77
  single brain metastasis, 77–78
  surgical technique, 79–81
  technological role in, 84–85
Bromodeoxyuridine (BUdR), 103
Burkitt's lymphoma, 159, 171

Calvarial metastasis, 118–119
Cancer related fatigue (CRF), 222–223, 230
Carboplatin-based therapy, 190–193
CD44, 12
Cellular adhesion molecules (CAMs), 9, 12
  Cerebral blood flow (CBF), 11, 42, 59

Cerebral blood volume (CBV), 33, 42, 46, 59, 122
Cerebrospinal fluid analysis, 174
Cervical cancer, 192
Chemotherapy, 177, 185
  concurrent, radiotherapy and, 216–217
  cutaneous malignancies and, 192–193
  dose-intensive, 177–178
  gynecologic malignancies and, 189–192
  interstitial, 106
  metastatic breast cancer and, 187–200
  multiagent, 203–206
  pre-radiation, 206
  responsiveness , 186
  single agent, 201–203
  temozolomide, 105–106
Chloromas, 170
Choriocarcinoma, see Gestational trophoblastic disease (GTD
Clear Cell Sarcoma of Kidney (CCSK), 155
CNS metastases
  diagnosis of, 173–174
  isolated, 174–175
  mechanisms for, 171–172
  treatment of, 175–176
Computed axial tomography (CT), 34–35, 129
Concurrent chemotherapy, radiotherapy and, 206–207
Contrast-enhanced CT (CECT), 34
Convection-enhanced delivery (CED), 87
Corticosteroids, in MBT patients, 58–60
Cranial nerve palsies, 132
Craniotomy, 84, 94, 221
Creatinine phosphokinase (CPK), 218
Crisis-intervention-oriented psychotherapy, 65
Cutaneous malignancies, 192–193Cytarabine, 172, 176

Deep venous thrombosis, 60–62
  prophylaxis for, 86
Dexamethasone, 58–60, 122
Diagnostic and Statistical Manual of Mental Disorders III (DSM III), 63–68
Diffuse large B-cell lymphoma (DLBCL), 170
Diffusion tensor imaging (DTI), 39
Diffusion weighted imaging (DWI), 38–39

Doxorubicin/cyclophosphamide/taxane
    therapy, 187
Dural metastases (DM)
    clinical findings for, 119–121
    epidemiology, 117–118
    diagnosis and, 121–122
    pathophysiology, 118–119
    prognosis for, 122
    radiological diagnosis of, 121–122
    treatment for, 122
DVT, *see* Deep venous thrombosis
Dysphagia and swallowing disorders, 62–63

E-cadherin, epithelial cadherin, 9, 10
Efaproxiril (RSR-13), 104–105
Electroencephalography (EEG), 56
Electromyogram (EMG) testing, 218
EMA/CO therapy, 191
Endometrial cancer, chemotherapy and, 191–192
Endothelial addressins, 12
Epidermal growth factor (EGF), 13
Epidermal growth factor receptor (EGFR), 188
Epithelial-mesenchymal transition (EMT), 7
Epithelial ovarian cancer, chemotherapy and,
    189 190
Epoeitinalfa (EPO), 222
Estrogen receptor (ER), 186
Ewing's sarcoma, 145–146
Extracellular matrix (ECM), 9–10, 12

Fallopian tube cancer, chemotherapeutic
    management for, 190
FDG-6-phosphate, 45
FDG-PET, 34, 45, 122
    scanning, 122
Fluid-attenuated inversion recovery
    (FLAIR), 174
Focal treatment, 107–110
    WBRT with, 94

Gamma Knife® radiosurgery, 27–28, 95
Gasserian ganglion syndrome, 125–127
Gastric acid inhibitors, MBT patients and, 60
Germ cell tumors, 151–152
    of ovary, chemotherapy for, 151–152
Gestational trophoblastic disease (GTD), 185, 191
Gliadel^{TM}, 86
Glutamine, 55
Gradient recalled echo (GRE), 33, 39, 43, 45
    imaging, 38–39

Gynecologic malignancies, chemotherapy and
    cervical cancer, 192
    endometrial cancer, 191–192
    fallopian tube cancer, 190
    germ cell tumors of ovary, 190
    gestational trophoblastic disease, 191
    ovarian cancer, 189–190

Hematologic malignancies, brain metastases in,
    169–170
    chemotherapy, dose-intensive, 177–178
    CNS prophylaxis, 172
    non-Hodgkin's lymphoma, CNS involvement
        in, 171–172
Heparan sulfate proteoglycans (HSPG), 12
Hepatoblastoma, 149–150
HER2/neu status, metastatic breast cancer
    and, 187
Hodgkin's lymphoma, 159–160
Human epidermal growth factor receptor, 2
    (HER-2), 4
Hypofractionated stereotactic radiotherapy
    (HSRT), 26–27
Hypoxic ischemic factor (HIF), 13–14

Incidence, of brain metastases
    in children, 5
    from specific cancers, 3–5
Infiltrating ductal carcinoma histology (IDC), 186
INI1 gene, 156
Integrin-linked kinase (ILK), 10
International Lymphoma Study Group
    (ILSG), 170
International Primary CNS Lymphoma
    Collaborative Group (IPCG), 175
International Prognostic Index (IPI)
    classification, 172
Interstitial chemotherapy, 106
Iodomethyltyrosine (IMT), SPECT and, 45

Jugular foramen syndrome, 127

Karnofsky Performance Status (KPS), 64,
    106, 218
    depression and, 64

Lactate dehydrogenase (LDH), 171
Lapatinib, 189
Leptomeningeal carcinomatosis, 117, 118
Leptomeningeal metastases, 173–174, 176

Level of alertness (LOA), in symptomatic
    patients, 62–63
Levetiracetam, in brain tumor patients, 67
Locoregional therapy, 86–87
Low-molecular-weight heparin (LMWH), 61,
    86, 221–222

Magnetic resonance imaging, 31, 35–37, 80,
    129, 173–174, 186, 206
    diffusion tensor imaging, 39–42
    diffusion weighted imaging, 38–9
    DM diagnosis and, 121
    GRE imaging, 38–39
    MR spectroscopy, 43, 121
    perfusion imaging, 42, 44
    post-contrast T1 weighted imaging, 39–42
    T1–weighted imaging, 37, 42
    T2/FLAIR imaging, 37–38
Magnetization-prepared rapid gradient echo
    (MP-RAGE), 129
Magnetization transfer, 42
Malignant melanoma, 152–153
Malignant rhabdoid tumor of kidney (MRTK),
    155–156
Matrix metalloproteins (MMPs), 10, 12
MBT patients, see Metastatic brain tumors
    patients
Meningioma, DM diagnosis, 121
Mental neuropathy,see Numb chin
    syndrome (NCS)
Merkel cell carcinoma (MCC), 192–193
Metastatic brain tumors patients,symptom
    management and supportive care of,
    53–56
    anticoagulation, thromboembolic
        complications and, 60–62
    corticosteroids, 58–60
    gastric acid inhibitors, 60
    psychiatric issues, 63–68
    role of, 54
    seizures and anticonvulsant therapy, 55–58
    swallowing disorders, dysphagia and,
        62–63
Metastatic breast cancer, chemotherapy and,
    187–189
"Metastatic cascade", 8, 9
    adhesion, 12
    angiogenesis, 13–14
    colonization, 12–13
    detachment, 9
    extravasation, 12
        intravasation, 9–10
        transport and embolization, 10–11
Micrometastases, 12–14
Middle fossa syndrome, see Gasserian ganglion
    syndrome
Misonidazole, 103
MMP-2, 10
MMP-9, 10
Molecular recognition hypothesis, 8
Motexafin gadolinium (MGd), 91, 103
MRI, see Magnetic resonance imaging
MR spectroscopy (MRS), 43–44, 121
Multiagent chemotherapy, 201, 203–206
Multiple brain metastases, 78–79

National Comprehensive Cancer Network
    (NCCN), 222, 224
National Institute of Neurological and
    Communicative Disorders and Stroke
    (NINCDS), 2
National Wilm's Tumor Study Group studies
    (NWTS), 154–156
N-cadherin, neuronal cadherin, 9
Neuroblastoma (NB), 150–151
Neurocognitive and physical disability, in brain
    metastatic patient
    end of life issues, hospice care and, 225–226
    ethical issues, 227–228
Neurocognitive function, in patient with brain
    metastases, 100–102
Neuroimaging
    computed axial tomography (CT), 34–35
    magnetic resonance imaging, 35–37,
        80, 129
    nuclear medicine, 34, 42, 44
Neuro-radiologic imaging, 173–174
NHL, see Non-Hodgkin's lymphoma
N-MYC oncogene amplification, 150
Non-Hodgkin's lymphoma, 159
    CNS involvement in, 170–171
    CNS prophylaxis in patients with, 172
    CNS relapse of, 177–178
    as isolated disease, 174–175
    leptomeningeal metastases and, 173–4
Non-small cell lung cancer (NSCLC), 201, 203,
    206–207
North American Brain Tumor Coalition, 54
Numb chin syndrome (NCS), 128

Occipital condyle syndrome consists, 128
Ommaya reservoir, 176

Orbital syndrome, 124–125
Osteosarcoma, 146–147

Pachymeningitis carcinomatosa, 129, *see also*
    Dural metastases (DM)
Palliative care, for brain metastatic patients
    AEDs, use of, 220–221
    steroid side effects, 216–220
    steroid treatment, 215–216
    supportive care issues, 222–229
    venous thromboembolism, 221–222
Parasellar syndrome, 125
Parenchymal brain metastases
    epidemiology, 31–32
    neuroimaging *see* Neuroimaging
    pathophysiology, imaging correlates and,
        32–33
    post-treatment evaluation, 46
    presentation, 32
    solitary lesion, 45–46
    steroids and, 46
    T2 hypointensity in, 33, 37–38
Parenchymal metastatic lesions, 32–34
Pathophysiology, of brain metastases, 5–6
    BBB and, 14–15
    CNS lymphatics and, 15
    "metastatic cascade" *see* "Metastatic cascade"
    metastatic cell, 6–7
    microenvironment, 7–8
Pediatric brain metastasis, extraneural
        malignancies and, 143–160
    leukemia, 156–159
    lymphoma, 156, 159–160
    renal tumors, 153–155
    solid tumors, 144–153
Perfusion imaging, 42–43
Peripheral neuroectodermal tumor (PNET),
    145, 156
Peritumoral edema, corticosteroids and, 58–60
PET/CT scan, 130
Platelet derived growth factor (PDGF), 13
Pneumocystis carinii pneumonia (PCP), 60
Pneumocystis jirovecii pneumonia (PJP),
    216–217
Positron emission tomography (PET), 3, 44
    scanning, 3, 42, 122
Pre-radiation chemotherapy, 206–207
Psychiatric issues, MBT patients and, 63–68
Psychotherapy, 65
Pulmonary embolism (PE), 60–61

Radiation Therapy Oncology Group (RTOG), 77,
    92–93, 95–96, 104–105
Radiation therapy, skull base metastasis and,
    130–132
Radiation Treatment Oncology Group recursive
    portioning analysis (RTOG RPA), 199
Radiolabeled fluorodeoxyglucose (FDG), 45
Radionuclide scans, 129–130
Radiosensitizers, 103
Radiosurgery, 23–24
    versus surgical resection, 24–27
    and WBRT, 95–96
Radiotherapy, concurrent chemotherapy and,
    206–207
Recursive partitioning analysis (RPA)
    classification, 77, 92–93, 122
Renal tumors
    clear cell sarcoma of kidney, 155
    rhabdoid tumor of kidney, 155–156
    Wilm's tumor, 153–154
Resection, 97–98
    and WBRT, 94–95
Retinoblastoma, 148–149
Rhabdomyosarcoma, 147–148
Rituximab-CHOP chemotherapy (R-CHOP),
    170, 178

Satellite tumor, 7–8
Seizures and anticonvulsant therapy, in MBT
    patients, 65–68
Sellar syndrome, 138–139
Serotonin specific reuptake inhibitor (SSRI), 77
Single agent chemotherapy, 211–213
Single brain metastasis, 87–88
Single photon emission computed tomography
    (SPECT), 49
    with radiolabeled amino acids, 52
    scans, 140
Skull-base metastasis
    diagnosis of, 139–140
    gasserian ganglion syndrome, 135–137
    jugular foramen syndrome, 137
    numb chin syndrome (NCS), 138
    occipital condyle syndrome, 138
    orbital syndrome, 134–135
    parasellar syndrome, 135
    pathophysiology, 133
    prognosis of, 142
    sellar syndrome, 138–139
    temporal bone syndrome, 137–138
    treatment of, 140–142

Small cell lung cancer (SCLC), 211, 213, 216

Solitary lesion, 54–55

MR perfusion and, 46

Sphenocavernous sinus metastasis, *see* Parasellar
syndrome

Spin echo (SE), 36, 46

Stereotactic radiosurgery (SRS), 92, 105,
132, 142

Stereotactic surgical navigation device, 94

Steroid myopathy, 228

Steroids, 55–56

treatment, in brain metastatic patient, 225–226

Steroid side effects

CNS side effects, 228–229

pneumocystis jirovecii pneumonia, 226–227

steroid myopathy, 228

Supratentorial tumors, seizures and, 65

Surgery, technological role in, 94–95

Surgical resection *versus* radiosurgery, 24–27

Surgical technique, brain metastases and, 89–91

Surveillance Epidemiology and End Results
(SEER), 1, 169

Swallowing disorders and dysphagia, in MBT
patients, 72–73

T1 mapping, 45

T1-weighted imaging, 36, 139

post-contrast, 41–44

T-1 weighted gadolinium images, 184

T2-FLAIR imaging, 36–38

T2-weighted images, 131

Technitium 99m methoxyisobutylisonitrile
(^{99m}Tc MIBI), 51–52

Temozolomide (TMZ), 115–116, 211–212,
216–217

Temporal bone syndrome, 137–138

Thallium-201 (^{201}Tl) SPECT, 49–51

Three dimensional gradient echo (3D GE), 42, 54

Thromboembolism and anticoagulation, in brain
tumor patients, 70–72

Tissue factor (TF), 11

TMZ, *see* Temozolomide (TMZ)

Trastuzumab, 197–198

Trilateral retinoblastoma (TRb), 159

Trimethoprim-sulphamethoxazole
(TMP-SMX), 70

TrkB, anti-apoptotic molecule, 10

Tumor-associated seizures (TAS), 65

Two dimensional spin echo (2D SE), 42

UPA-uPAR complex, 12

Urokinase plasminogen activator (uPA), 10

Urokinase plasminogen activator receptor
(uPAR), 10

Vascular endothelial growth factor (VEGF), 13,
68–69

Vena cava filter (VCF), 71–72

Venous thromboembolism (VTE), 231–232

WAGR syndrome, 163

Whole Brain Radiation Therapy(WBRT), 76, 77,
78, 79, 91, 92–107, 122, 185, 189–192, 223

adjuvant, utility of, 109–110, 132

complications of, 104

dose and schedule, 103–104

radiosurgery and, 105–106

resection and, 104–105

resection *vs.* radiosurgery and, 106–107

Wilm's tumor, 163–164